THE
EXERCISE PLUS

PRE

DATE DUE

THE
EXERCISE PLUS
PREGNANCY
PROGRAM

Exercises for Before,
During, and After Pregnancy

by
Lazar and Olinda Cedeno
and Carole Monroe

Photographs by Laura Beaujon

WILLIAM MORROW AND COMPANY, INC.
New York   1980

Library of Congress Cataloging in Publication Data

Cedeno, Lazar.
   The exercise plus pregnancy program.

   "Morrow quill paperbacks."

   1. Prenatal care.   2. Exercise for women.
3. Pregnancy.   4. Postnatal care.   I. Cedeno,
Olinda, joint author.   II. Monroe, Carole, joint
author.   III. Title.
RG558.7.C42   1980b   618.2'4   80-14280
ISBN 0-688-03697-X
ISBN 0-688-08697-7 (pbk.)

Printed in the United States of America

First Morrow Quill Paperback Edition

1   2   3   4   5   6   7   8   9   10

BOOK DESIGN BY MICHAEL MAUCERI

*For expectant and newly delivered mothers everywhere
who are discovering or rediscovering the joy of pregnancy*

Foreword

The first baby I ever delivered as a young medical student is now voting age. The baby was born of a young unconscious mother who had been sedated heavily and then anesthetized. She would not be totally aware of her new daughter until an hour after delivery. The baby was also quite sleepy at birth and required careful watching and some assistance with breathing. The traditional elation associated with a new life was dulled by the fatigued, experienced physicians around me as they routinely went about the task of bringing both mother and newborn back to consciousness. Although not exactly what I had thought it would be, it was still my first delivery. Since "firsts" in one's life are very special, my pulse raced and my heart was full. In fact, I had probably sponged up that delivery room's entire allotment of thrill and pride and joy, including the very large portion that should have appropriately gone to the new mother and father.

Fortunately, the obstetrical world has changed since the birth of that baby almost two decades ago. In part, the change was in response to the heightened and sophisticated demands of a more enlightened group of new parents. The change was also due to the inevitable ladder of medical scientific advances and the accumulation and interpretation of large bodies of statistical data.

One thing that doctors and patients have come to agree upon strongly is that sleepy babies born of unconscious mothers (not as a necessity but as a routine gesture) are statistically less likely to become intellectual leaders in our society.

During the 1960's and 1970's, the obstetrical research centers underwent a mini-revolution. The uterus can now be scrutinized by a fetoscope or by ultrasound (sonography), and its fluid sampled by needle tap (amniocentesis). It is now routinely possible to determine fetal lung maturity and, therefore, readiness for birth, and to forestall or even stop premature labor so as to extend intrauterine life and maturity when medically wise.

Yet, ironically, one of the greatest advances in modern childbearing and birthing was not an increase in the sophistication of technical apparatus, but rather a "throw-back," a full-cycle return to a simpler day.

I speak of a new era of family participation in which the mother and father are as aware and present during pregnancy and birthing as they were during conception, where medical science intervenes only when necessary, and fewer and fewer prospective parents are awed or frightened by their obstetrician or midwife, or by the process of childbirth itself. Because of discussion in the media, increased higher education, the tendency to start a family at a more mature age, and open discussion of things formerly just not talked about—for all these reasons, mystery is no longer fashionable in obstetrics and childbearing.

The prospective mother's role is once again an active one. More and more she is tolerating minor symptoms rather than ingesting drugs for their alleviation, in order to insure maximum purity in her unborn baby's environment. The father's role is also much more involved. The prospective father is present in the examining room with the expectant mother. Both ask questions, and often take turns supporting and encouraging one another during the pregnancy. Fathers are distinctly part of the process.

In all fairness, however, it is not the prospective father's body that undergoes change. It is in the realm of body change and body image that childbearing remains totally and uniquely a woman's experience. The physical change is real. Her breasts and abdomen enlarge, and her center of gravity changes. There is an additional strain on her lower back, and muscles never used even casually are now overtaxed. While some women may suffer a myriad of unpleasant physical symptoms, others may be more fortunate. One's comfort during pregnancy cannot be guaranteed solely because of physical fitness, but I do believe that those whose muscles are limber and frequently used will find pregnancy easier, and will recapture their vigor and pre-pregnancy shape far more easily and rapidly.

I feel strongly that proper exercises will help to maintain a woman's body image and physical confidence. It is not sufficient simply to take a natural childbirth course, which really is geared to those last hours of pregnancy, emphasizing only those muscles that aid in pushing the baby out, or in tightening the vaginal muscles to alleviate episiotomy discomfort. It is the preceding thirty-eight weeks that have likely strengthened or destroyed the new mother's concept of self, and it is without question in the post-partum period that an ounce of prevention is worth a pound of care in terms of muscle tautness and weight control.

This book will, if used properly, increase the tone of a pregnant woman's body and activate muscles last used far too long ago. Obviously, the degree and extent of this improvement will be dependent on individual variations and on an adherence to the regime itself. The book will take study. It will likely evolve into a narrator-exercise format, with the prospective father as narrator—another rather lovely thing to do together during pregnancy. In addition, the rewards of muscle control, relaxation, and breathing control will indeed augment and not conflict with the subsequent natural and prepared childbirth courses taken by most new parents today.

I have read the book and will surely recommend it to my patients. There are, no doubt, exceptional individuals who for cardiac or other medical reasons should not exercise during pregnancy. I would advise all prospective users of this book to seek the approval of their physicians before embarking on the program.

I congratulate the authors on their book. It fulfills a most dramatic need at a time when any assistance, much less a book of this importance and value, should be appreciated and taken advantage of.

—NATHAN MANDELMAN, M.D., F.A.C.O.G.
Assistant Clinical Professor of Obstetrics
and Gynecology
Mount Sinai School of Medicine
New York, N. Y.

Acknowledgments

We wish to mutually acknowledge and thank Maria Carvainis and Bob Bender for their encouragement, support, and enthusiasm for this project.

Special thanks and appreciation go to Elisabeth Bing, whose pioneering efforts in the natural childbirth field have made us all aware of the importance of being fit before, during, and after pregnancy.

Contents

Introduction

by Lazar Cedeno

How to keep in shape at a time when every woman feels most out of shape is the aim of the EXERCISE PLUS program. Whether you are planning to have a child, have just learned you are expecting, or are in your sixth to eighth month, your pregnancy and delivery will be easier the better you have prepared for it.

It is important to remember that your pregnancy is not an illness but a beautiful, normal, and natural state of being. It is a time in your life—and your man's life—that is meant to be enjoyed. In order to enjoy it, you will have to feel good. Good nutrition, a healthy mental state, and proper exercise will all contribute to your feeling of well-being, freeing you to enjoy life at a time when it is meant to be enjoyed to the fullest.

Working closely with your gynecologist, midwife, or team of experts, and staying in touch with what your body is telling you and showing you right now, will maximize your birth experience and help it go smoothly. Before embarking on any change in your normal daily routine—your diet or an exercise program, in particular—it is always wise to consult your physician first.

The EXERCISE PLUS program you are about to start is the

result of a cumulative forty years of experience working with the body, and was inspired by Olinda's pregnancy with our third child. We met when we were both professional dancers at the Dance Theater of Harlem. I had studied with many of the top choreographers in dance today, including George Balanchine, Anna Sokolow, and Peter Wright of the Royal Ballet. I had danced with the San Francisco Ballet and had performed with the New York City Ballet. Olinda had studied at the Harkness House for Ballet Arts and had also performed with the New York City Ballet.

We were married in 1972, and when Olinda became pregnant with our first child, we decided to leave ballet since the idea of touring with a family was not appealing. At that time a friend of ours, Richard Nickolaus, was just beginning his Nickolaus Exercise Centers, and he asked me to join him in managing one of his first studios in New York City. We became very involved with the development of the Nickolaus technique, but in 1975 left to start our own studio.

Olinda became active in the business, and even throughout her second pregnancy we worked closely together in developing and refining the exercises, and in teaching classes in our studio. Even though Olinda had been a dancer and had kept herself in shape during her first two pregnancies, it wasn't until her third that she adapted the exercises we were teaching in the studio to meet her special needs and those of other pregnant women. In January 1979, to meet the growing number of new clients, we set up regular classes exclusively for expectant and newly delivered mothers.

The idea caught on immediately, and the response to the expectant mothers' exercise classes was truly exciting for us. "I started feeling good about myself immediately," one of the women told us. "I had never really stuck to an exercise program, feared I was going to put on too much weight, and was aware from all I'd read that the actual labor and delivery would be quite a strenuous exercise in itself.

"I started EXERCISE PLUS in my fourth month. Right away a nagging lower backache I'd begun to suffer with eased up a great deal. My posture improved, I felt more relaxed about my pregnancy, and more in control of how I would feel and look over the next five months."

Nancy Cuddihy, a midwife at Roosevelt Hospital's very successful midwifery program, visited one of Olinda's classes and encouraged her to get more women involved in her exercise program. Over the years Nancy had noticed how much easier delivery is for an expectant mother who is in good physical shape.

"The very best side effect of exercise is relaxation and relief from anxiety," she says. "Of the more than three hundred and fifty women a year registered in the Roosevelt Hospital midwifery program, most are between twenty-eight and thirty years old, 80 percent have college degrees or better, and most are there because they want to maximize their birthing experience. While these women are learning all about delivery, they are also learning that the most important part of their delivery will be their breathing and relaxation."

The plus in our EXERCISE PLUS program is rhythmic breathing, which is what we stress in all our classes. We developed the rhythmic breathing technique after years of observing the breathing patterns of dancers doing warm-up exercises and training for performances. We were amazed to realize that with all the training that we as dancers went through, we were never taught to breathe properly. Most dancers and many athletes have a tendency to hold their breath while in motion and to pant when tired. Both reactions are out of sync with the natural order of things. Once we developed rhythmic breathing for use during exercise and training, we noticed immediate relief from tiredness, and our stamina and strength were restored.

One of the leading gynecologists at New York's Mt. Sinai Hospital made this observation about the benefits of slow, rhythmic breathing taught in our EXERCISE PLUS classes:

"Deep breathing, with an emphasis on slow rhythmicity, increases lung expansion, contraction, and relaxation. But it also goes further. It stimulates other muscles in the trunk and pelvic area, relaxing them more completely as well.

"By coordinating deep breathing with physical exercise, you are getting a much larger quantity of oxygen into your system and getting rid of more carbon dioxide residue than you normally do. This helps the muscles to work more efficiently because they are well aerated. With muscles working at their maximum, your body feels stronger and can work out longer without getting so tired.

"The benefits of rhythmic breathing are going to be most appreciated during labor. The time between contractions becomes minimal, and unless you can totally relax body muscles, enabling your body to rid itself of waste and to catch up with itself in terms of energy and metabolism, you'll be one haggard and exhausted patient."

Nancy Cuddihy told us that some of the most impressive deliveries she has seen are the ones in which a woman is successful at "letting go." These women "seem to flow with the labor," she says. "The baby just passes through their body, and there is no holding back. Basically the birth canal is a muscle that has to open and stretch. If you are relaxed, the muscle is not going to be so rigid or tense. It's like putting your head through the neckline of a very tight T-shirt—you want it to soften and open wide in order to get through."

Exercise, plus breathing, will play an important part, then, in helping you feel refreshed, relaxed, and yet invigorated at a time when you would more often feel bulky, sore, and stiff. Successfully completing an exercise program will give you a greater sense of control over your body. Being in control, while at the same time being relaxed, will give you the confidence and trust you'll need to "let go" for a smoother labor and delivery.

We assume that since you have this book, you are at least considering or are already committed to an exercise program. Because this childbearing year is such a crucial one for you, you have even more incentive to exercise than the average woman who may just have decided that it would be a good thing for her to do. In fact, no matter how late in your pregnancy you may now be, consider this: It is far better to begin exercising today than to undertake one of the most strenuous exercises of all—your labor and delivery—in an out-of-shape condition.

There are virtually no exercises in the EXERCISE PLUS program that are anywhere near as strenuous as your actual labor and delivery will be. But if you are still a little uncomfortable with the idea of exercise during pregnancy, you should feel safer and more relaxed about it after you've consulted your gynecologist and read through this book.

According to *The U.S. Air Force Academy Fitness Program for Women* by Jack Galub (New Jersey: Prentice-Hall, 1979):

> There is little question that pregnancy is no handicap to the active woman. . . . Still the odds are that few obstetricians will permit a deconditioned pregnant woman suddenly to undertake vigorous exercise. If she has been active, there

should be little reason for her not continuing as long as there is no danger of injuring her back or falling.

In the EXERCISE PLUS program for expectant mothers, there is virtually no possibility of your falling, since all but the last few exercises are done on a mat on the floor. And from beginning to end, your back is one of the major areas that will benefit from each and every exercise. With our emphasis on strengthening abdominal muscles, you will find that your spine is getting the support that is so necessary to protect it during childbearing.

No part of the body will be exercised without being properly warmed up first. This is very important because a warmed-up muscle is one that is protected from injury. It is more relaxed and therefore less likely to undergo undue stress or strain. Keeping this in mind, we begin our program with exercises that get the blood flowing, relax you, and warm you up in every area of your body, from head to toe.

From a simple neck stretch to rhythmic foot circles, we move on to more strenuous exercises, increasing the blood flow to each area as we work your body in a systematic, sequential order—legs, trunk, pelvis, and arms. Then we have you on your feet for the last set of exercises, which will leave your body in perfect alignment, prepared for whatever the rest of your day has in store.

It is important, and we will remind you of this throughout the book, that you completely master each exercise before going on to the next. As we explained above, we've designed the entire program with a special order in mind, so that it is essential you perform the exercises in the sequence presented.

We'd like to suggest before going any further that you turn to Chapter 3 and take a look through the exercise program. We have written each routine and illustrated it with photographs that will allow you to visually understand the rhythm of your movements. On reading the text, you will grasp the principles behind each exercise so that even without an instructor, you will execute them correctly.

Then, even before you begin your first exercise, it is very important that you take some quiet moments to sit and read the book all the way through. In the next two chapters we go into detail about the changes your body will go through during the childbearing year and afterward, and we explain further just how and why the EXERCISE PLUS program works.

We feel that the more you know about your body right now, the more incentive you will have to begin and maintain a regular program. You are fortunate to have a very strong incentive to exercise right now because you are or may soon be pregnant. In fact, you may find that even if you were active and have exercised before, you may not have been as consistent as you will probably be now. Many of our students have told us, "Being pregnant is motivation enough to be regular about exercising."

You are also fortunate to have selected the EXERCISE PLUS program, and we say this honestly and proudly. We see the results of the program every day in our classes, and our students also see the results every time they look in the mirror.

The real beauty of the program is that it works. You immediately notice the improvements. And each time you exercise, you feel your body responding as it becomes stronger and firmer.

You will get a great deal of pleasure from seeing and feeling the results of your efforts so quickly. This pleasure will only reinforce your already strong motivation for exercising, making it easier and easier to maintain a regular routine two to three hours a week.

Proper exercise and diet will enhance your pregnancy and birth experience. By following the EXERCISE PLUS program, with its emphasis on rhythmic breathing, you will be able to flow with your labor and delivery because you will have trained your body well. And you will have kept your body fit so that after delivery, you can more easily regain your most desirable shape.

Chapter 1

How and Why the EXERCISE PLUS Program Works

▼▼

As your pregnancy progresses, your muscles will stretch, your ligaments soften, and your joints loosen in order to accommodate the growing baby. If your muscles are toned, they will provide the structural support your body needs to accommodate these changes.

If they are not toned—and unfortunately that is the case for the vast majority of women—your pregnancy will add additional stress to these supporting muscles. This means that certain areas of your body—in particular the pelvic floor muscles, the abdomen, and the backbone—could weaken to the point of becoming troublesome. These are the areas we concentrate on in EXERCISE PLUS.

What we'd like to emphasize is that at this time your need for exercise has gone beyond that of just wanting to get in shape, and to maintain and quickly restore your figure. Your need now is to be in shape throughout your pregnancy and afterward in order to avoid unnecessary, though often common, problems such as backache, loss of urinary control, hemorrhoids, discomfort in intercourse, and lack of pelvic organ support.

You'll want your muscles to be strong enough to protect your back. As your abdomen stretches and the baby's weight increases, the curve in your backbone increases, and your whole center of gravity moves slightly forward.

Without strong muscular support, this can result in your pelvis tilting forward as well, and your posture is sure to be poor. Poor posture on anyone, but particularly on a pregnant woman, is a direct cause of fatigue and backache.

You'll need your abdominal muscles to be strong and under your control to help protect your back as well. As these muscles stretch, if they are allowed to weaken due to neglect, you'll wind up with not only a flabby, floppy belly but an added strain on a backbone that needs all the support it can get.

And you'll want all your voluntary muscles to be well toned for the time when you'll need them the most—during delivery. In childbirth, good strong muscles must function smoothly, as you need them for coordination and relaxation to allow the uterus to work freely in the birth process. Remember, after only six weeks the uterus will return to its original state because on its own it will continue involuntary contractions. Only you—by exercising your abdominal muscles—can return them to their desired size and function after delivery.

If you are aware of any potential weaknesses or problems that may arise due to lack of exercise, you'll be able to reverse or correct them with the program we've designed. You are just not going to be able to adequately exercise the key muscles involved in childbearing during your normal activities. Even if you are a sportswoman, a runner, or a walker, you will still have to concentrate on properly exercising your back, pelvic area, and abdomen.

Developing good posture will be one of your major goals, so that your body can carry the load of pregnancy. Fortunately it is one of the primary benefits of the EXERCISE PLUS program. Almost immediately you will learn how to align parts of your body, in whatever position you assume, so that your joints and muscles are protected from strain.

Developing and maintaining strong abdominal muscles will be another major goal. Practically every exercise in the program will work your stomach, so that from the beginning we will be concentrating on this area for maximum support of the pelvic floor.

The Plus in EXERCISE PLUS: Rhythmic Breathing

Now is a good time to explain fully what we mean by rhythmic breathing and how it works.

Our technique is based on the natural way to breathe when your body is in a completely relaxed state. You breathe in, and as your lungs fill with air, your stomach expands; breathe out, your stomach flattens. One of the very first exercises you will be doing is the breathing exercise—lying flat on your back, knees up, hands on your stomach, you will inhale on two counts and exhale on two counts— which sets the rhythmic pattern you will maintain throughout the program. This rhythmic breathing is the key to relaxation. Knowing how to relax will enhance your chances for a successful labor and delivery.

There are two ways to breathe when undergoing an activity— a right way and a wrong way. Below is an example of the wrong way to breathe, and, unfortunately, it is the way most of us breathe, especially when exerting ourselves.

Picture a man lifting a heavy box. You can see him take in a deep breath, hold it in as he squats to lift the box, and get red in the face as he exerts his entire body in the process of lifting that box. Sweat begins to pop out all over his face, his veins engorge with blood, and exhaustion sets in.

The correct way for this man to have undertaken this stressful activity would have been to breathe in deeply in preparation for lifting the heavy box, then to exhale, contracting his abdominal muscles, and to continue breathing rhythmically while executing the rest of the action.

It is so crucial to breathe correctly while exercising that we can't emphasize it enough. In fact, we will tell you during each exercise when to breathe in and when to breathe out.

It might help if you imagine your torso—your abdomen and chest —as a balloon. You, the balloon, are the recipient of oxygen. As you breathe in fully, your abdomen and chest areas fill up with air until they can't get any fuller. As you breathe out, the reverse takes place, and you, the balloon, shrink as the chest and abdomen deflate. To completely empty your balloon of all air, you force it out by pulling and squeezing in your abdominal muscles until there is no air left.

This correct breathing technique becomes rhythmic when it is coupled with the exercises. All our exercises are coordinated with the same breathing pattern: You breathe in deeply for two counts and breathe out fully for two counts. As you inhale on two counts, you fill your body with air. As you exhale on two counts, you flatten your abdomen and chest against your spine. These abdominal contractions that accompany the expulsion of the breath are the preparation for each and every exercise you will be doing.

As Elizabeth Noble explains in her book *Essential Exercises for the Childbearing Year* (Boston: Houghton Mifflin, 1976), remember to "breathe in as you stretch, extend, lift up, or move the body backward; breathe out as you return to starting position, or to a forward or flex position. Breathe out when contracting the abdominal muscles."

It is one of the major aims of the EXERCISE PLUS program that correct breathing techniques become so well developed you will automatically breathe this way all the time, not just while we're reminding you to. After a while, correct breathing will become second nature to you. If you receive no other benefit from doing the EXERCISE PLUS exercises regularly, you will learn to breathe correctly no matter what position you're in or activity you engage in.

Instead of holding your breath tight in moments of high energy —a reflex action that most of us have—you will take in air in preparation for a movement and let it out as you perform the movement.

It is especially important for you to develop good breathing habits during pregnancy. As pressure in the abdomen increases with the growth of your baby, respiratory muscle movement decreases, which can often cause discomfort and congestion.

Coordinating your movements during exercise with deep rhythmic breathing will ensure that your entire system will receive the greatest amount of oxygen. As you inhale deeply, filling your lungs with air, the air will enter the farthest recesses of the lungs, where the actual exchange of oxygen and carbon dioxide takes place.

When you're exercising, two things are happening at once. You are expending more energy, and in turn burning fat and carbohydrates to make more energy. The energy that is released during exercise makes your blood flow faster, so that your muscles receive more blood and in turn can more quickly get rid of the waste they produce when at work. It is the accumulation of waste, the toxins, that causes tired, stiff muscles.

Of course, an increased blood flow stimulates muscle fibers, so that they become stronger and work more efficiently. Since women don't produce the hormone testosterone, which men do, their muscles don't develop in exercise as men's do, but rather improve in tone. Besides, the EXERCISE PLUS exercises were carefully worked out so that they do not bunch up the muscles and do not form unsightly bulges. Instead, the emphasis is on tone and conditioning, on stretching and strengthening.

The increased oxygen flow will also aerate the muscles, so that you won't become red in the face as you exert yourself. Your blood circulation will improve greatly. Since the main vein from the lower limbs, abdomen, and pelvis passes through the diaphragm, the pumping action from rhythmic breathing speeds up the blood flow and improves circulation throughout the body. And even though you will be working hard during these exercises, you won't even perspire very much.

The fact is that while you are executing your EXERCISE PLUS routines, when you breathe properly, you are simultaneously exercising your entire body. Just mastering rhythmic breathing so that it becomes the natural way to breathe all the time will mean an increase in energy and an overall improvement in your physical and mental well-being.

Along with the surge of oxygen provided by rhythmic breathing you will experience a vital flow of energy into all your muscles that will give you the stamina you will need to repeat the exercises. At the same time, the oxygen flow will keep your body relaxed, so that you only tighten the specific muscle area you are working on.

We emphasize slow rhythmic breathing because if you take too many quick deep breaths in succession, you can get dizzy. Shallow breathing could lead to breathlessness after only mild exertion. Holding your breath during exercise can result in exhaustion. And muscles and tissues deprived of oxygen while being exercised will be achy and tired afterward.

You may feel an overall tiredness after your workouts, but at the same time you will also feel stimulated and invariably more relaxed than when you began. Evidence keeps mounting that exercise executed with proper breathing not only produces beneficial physical changes but emotional ones as well. As Jack Galub says in *The U.S. Air Force Academy Fitness Program for Women:*

> To coin a cliché, fitness is in. Every day, it seems, more women are deciding they should exercise. . . . If a woman has guidance and is not overly deconditioned, her efforts may open new vistas of self-confidence and health. She can become a happier, more secure person.

Since the brain also needs oxygen to function well, and since exercise increases the blood flow, which brings oxygen to and removes waste from the brain, prolonged exercise with proper breathing maximizes the nutrients the brain will receive. This can cause chemical changes in the brain, so that feelings of mental alertness, uplift from depression, release from tension, and general well-being can result.

Joan, a regular client in our EXERCISE PLUS program for expectant mothers, told us happily after her first two months, "Besides physically feeling so much better in my second trimester than I had expected to, I also feel better about myself psychologically. I have a demanding job, which I love. But at the end of the day, I'm often tense from stress at work. One hour working out with Lazar's exercises brings me more tension release, body strength, and sense of accomplishment and confidence than any other physical activity I've undertaken."

A woman who is totally fit can easily be noticed, Jack Galub points out:

> She carries herself easily, erect. She has a smooth, quick walk. She is confident. . . . Her regular exercise accelerates the flow of nutrients and oxygen-carrying blood to every part of her body. It is this oxygen that some physiologists believe helps slow the aging process. Age we must, but exercise helps us pass through the years more gracefully by keeping our cardiovascular systems at high levels of efficiency and our bodies strong and flexible.

These benefits alone may be incentive enough so that on a day when you can feel yourself hesitating before beginning your EXERCISE PLUS regime, just the memory of how good you will feel afterward can get you going. Remind yourself that each and every exercise session improves your entire musculatory and circulatory systems (and firms up those thighs and buttocks!). Remember how much stronger yet graceful you are becoming, how relaxed yet exhilarated you feel, and pretty soon your body will begin to crave the exercises.

Students have told us, and we know from experience, that their EXERCISE PLUS routine is a gentle addiction, and if they go more than a few days without doing the exercises, their bodies demand that shot of good feeling they get after each session.

How the EXERCISE PLUS Program Works the Pelvic Floor

Just as everything else softens and loosens as your pregnancy progresses, so do the muscles in the pelvic floor. As part of practically every exercise in our program, we will be telling you to tighten your buttocks, squeeze your thighs together, and pull in your stomach as much as you can. These activities, as well as Exercise 10, The Pelvic Tilt, and Exercise 17, The Pelvic Stretch, will keep your pelvic floor muscles strong yet supple for maximum support of the growing uterus.

The importance of exercising these muscles is stressed in *Our Bodies, Ourselves* (Massachusetts: The Boston Women's Health Collective, 1972, 1976):

> Surrounding the vagina, urethra, and anus is a series of muscles called the pelvic floor muscles. These muscles are important for supporting lower organs. If these muscles are weak, are stretched unduly, or are cut during an improperly done episiotomy (in childbearing), cystocele (bladder falling into the vagina), prolapsed uterus (uterus falling into the vagina), or urinary incontinence (uncontrollable urination) can eventually occur. These complications are often corrected surgically, but could be prevented by knowing where the muscles are and strengthening them by contracting them voluntarily.

As Elisabeth Bing, the world-renowned childbirth expert, emphasizes in her book *Moving Through Pregnancy* (New York: Bantam Books, 1976), your

> pelvic floor muscles have to carry a great deal of added weight during pregnancy, and they also have to undergo a good amount of stretching while the baby is being born. If you strengthen those muscles through exercises well beforehand, the pelvic floor will become more elastic, which in turn means that it will support the weight of the baby better in pregnancy, it will stretch more easily during the birth of the child, and the area will return to its good and normal muscle tone in a very short time postpartum.

Exercise of the pelvic floor should take top priority, then, during pregnancy. Unfortunately, even in childbirth education classes, it is often neglected. Before going any further, it may be helpful for you to locate these muscles and learn to control them by doing a very simple exercise, the Kegel exercise.

While seated on a toilet, voluntarily start and then stop the urine flow several times. Let some urine out before beginning the exercise. Let a smaller amount pass each time you do the contraction.

This exercise illustrates your muscle power and control. The stopping and starting action works the sphincter muscles, the master muscles that encircle both the urethral and vaginal openings of the pelvic floor. Thus, when you tighten your front passage to stop urination, you are at the same time contracting and tightening the vagina.

You can do your Kegel exercise practically anywhere, not just while urinating, because no one can notice a thing. While sitting, standing or lying down, riding in a car, doing dishes, or relaxing in front of the TV, tighten the urethra in the same way you did to stop urinating. At the same time, tighten the vagina (you should feel this a little higher up and in the middle). Continue to hold the vagina and move farther upward to tighten the muscles in the rectum. Hold for a count of six, then release all the tension until you have relaxed to the limit.

You probably won't feel three distinct contractions, since the sphincter muscles seem to tighten spontaneously whenever one of them is tightened. Don't be concerned. The important thing is that you do the Kegel exercise many times over the course of each and every day. Start out doing it three times. Don't repeat it too often at first because the pelvic floor muscles will get tired. Build up your repetitions gradually, until you are doing the Kegel exercise around thirty times a day. We recommend you do this exercise in addition to our exercises. By the time you deliver, you will know very well how to tighten—and how to completely relax —the muscles that make up the pelvic floor.

As the gynecologist from Mt. Sinai Hospital stresses, "This ability to release the sphincters and pelvic floor tensions completely will be crucial during the second stage of labor, when you don't want to be pushing hard and tightening at the same time."

While you are going through your EXERCISE PLUS routine, you will be contracting then relaxing the muscles in your abdomen, thighs, and buttocks. These contractions will voluntarily draw up the pelvic floor, and the relaxations will return it to its horizontal position. You can increase the intensity and work this vital area harder by incorporating the Kegel exercise in your workout and by pretending to hold, then release, a penny between your buttocks.

Normally the pelvic floor is horizontal, but if it is unexercised, it may sag with the added pressure of pregnancy as the uterus begins to weigh more. Even day-to-day functions such as coughing, sneezing, lifting, running, laughing, and straining put pressure on this area.

When exercised, your pelvic floor muscles will provide all the support you will need. In addition—and here is an extra plus of our EXERCISE PLUS program—your vagina will become more snug. The vaginal muscles will improve in thickness and strength, and this can increase the pleasures of intercourse. After the stretching the vagina goes through during delivery, it is of the utmost importance to return it to its desired size and shape.

Because of the greater control you will have over the urethra, urinary incontinence (the leaking of urine) will probably not be a problem. Also, due to improved blood circulation in the area, you should have immediate relief from any pelvic congestion, and you should be able to avoid varicose veins in the vulva and rectum (hemorrhoids).

Another gynecologist we consulted talked about the importance of exercising the pelvic floor muscles, particularly in regard to preventing or minimizing varicose veins. "Pregnancy is a sitting duck situation for increased or enhanced varicosity," he told us. "Increased blood means increased flow of the blood that is pumped to the lower extremities; therefore, veins must work even harder to get this blood back.

"Also, as the uterus gets bigger, it will weigh down on veins of the pelvis which bring back a great deal of this blood from the lower extremities, and from the lower buttocks and anal area. It is more difficult for venous blood to return from lower extremities that are fighting against gravity to begin with. Having an additional fight getting by the fetus, which acts as a tourniquet by compressing these veins so that the blood has to be squeezed by, there is increased tendency toward varicosity."

He reminded us that varicose veins also can result from a familial predisposition, about which there is not much you can do, and from muscle tone, about which there is. Good muscle tone can act like a pair of hands, preventing veins from expanding. If the muscle and connective tissue around a vein is weakened, not toned, the vein stands a much greater chance of expanding, which results in hemorrhoids.

"Hemorrhoids, which are nothing more than varicosity, may occur because of increased iron intake," the doctor pointed out. "They may also result from pushing during the second stage of labor. Exercise of the pelvic area helps prevent hemorrhoids entirely or decreases their severity."

In summary: Just as in any other muscle group, the pelvic floor muscles respond to the demands made upon them, and progressive exercising will increase the size and power of each muscle fiber. Simultaneously, blood circulation will become more extensive, carrying more oxygen and nutrients to the muscles in the perineum, so that they will be elastic enough to stretch over the baby's head with minimal damage to muscle fibers. And, healthy and exercised, these muscles will be restored much sooner than those that have been neglected.

The EXERCISE PLUS Program Concentrates on Your Abdomen

Stomach or abdominal muscles are generally found to be the weakest group of muscles in our bodies. Their weakness is one of the most common causes of backache.

It may seem unlikely at first that muscles in the front of the body would have such a profound effect on pain and discomfort in the lower back area. However, their role is not only to support the pelvis but the spine as well.

Abdominal muscles are very complex and elaborate. They form an extensive four-way corset, spanning the front of the trunk from the breastbone and ribs to the pubic bones, and around the side of the pelvic ridge. This set of muscles works hard for us during many of our activities. Besides maintaining the proper positions of abdominal and pelvic organs, including the growing uterus, these muscles assist in breathing, coughing, and sneezing. They control the pelvic tilt, and help to flex, raise, rotate, and lower the trunk. They brace our body under such stresses as lifting and straining, and stabilize our lower back during leg raising.

Because they bear the responsibility for all this activity, it is imperative that the abdominal muscles be strong and firm. During pregnancy it is even more important to keep them in good shape so that they can adequately support the load in front, which is placing increasing stress on the backbone.

Care must be taken at this time to avoid positions or exercises that may further stretch your abdominal muscles. To emphasize the care that must be taken, we'd like to explain here what happens to these abdominal muscles in the childbearing year.

Along with all the other changes, the hormones circulating during pregnancy cause the central seam connecting the abdominal muscles to soften. Abdominal muscles and their seams are expanding and stretching to accommodate the growing baby. The recti muscles—the ones running vertically on each side of the central seam—bear the most stress from the pressure of the increasing weight of the baby.

Because of the stretching involved, these recti muscles may spread open at stress points along the way and even separate. Being in a lax or weak state makes them even more vulnerable to separation, particularly since strain during pregnancy and labor is registered along the central seam (just like a seam in clothing that is too tight). This strain could produce bulging in the abdominal wall. Once this happens, muscle imbalance and abdominal wall weakness may persist, resulting in poor posture and lower back pain.

To recapitulate: Your abdominal muscles are softening due to hormonal changes, stretching to accommodate an expanding uterus, and straining in later pregnancy and delivery while they are in their most vulnerable, elongated state. This is why it is so important to avoid positions and exercises that might cause additional separation of the recti muscles.

We understand the body and how it functions, and because the EXERCISE PLUS exercises are done on a mat on the floor (even by those who are not pregnant), they automatically prevent undue strain on joints and muscles, particularly the central abdominal seam.

To put your mind completely at ease before you begin the EXERCISE PLUS program, we'd like to point out right away that we don't do any exercises that would add stress to the abdomen. We completely avoid, for example, double leg raises. Instead, you will lift and lower one leg at a time, keeping the other leg bent. And we do not have you doing complete sit-ups and rollbacks until after delivery. Even during sit-ups after delivery, we avoid the old-fashioned posture of legs kept straight out front. We have you roll up and back slowly, knees bent, hands holding the thighs for support. Thus, we teach you to use your own body for leverage, and the force of gravity for resistance, whenever we have you raise and lower the trunk and legs. These facts, plus concentrating at all times on contracting the abdomen during exercise, protect it from stress and strain.

You will also notice as you look through Chapter 3 that we have excluded any exercise done while lying on the stomach. We wait to teach you these until after delivery, and so these exercises are outlined in Chapter 4. Exercises done while lying on the stomach would only add additional strain to your already stretching stomach muscles.

The abdominal muscles are not easy to strengthen. That is why we stress preliminary strengthening exercises, such as rhythmic breathing. When you exhale, you should completely empty your lungs, which will cause you to push your abdomen strongly against your spine. This abdominal contraction on exhaling will be part of each and every movement throughout the EXERCISE PLUS program.

In your childbirth preparation classes, you will be focusing on preparation for labor and delivery. By doing abdominal exercises —even if you are in your last trimester—you'll be able to maintain, strengthen, and firm up these crucial muscles. In turn, this will help you avoid unnecessary tension in the area. You'll be able to control and tighten, as well as relax, these muscles—an ability you'll need during delivery.

Well-exercised abdominal muscles become supple, and supple muscles—those that have maintained their contractile ability and blood circulation as much as possible—will lengthen more easily for delivery and will shorten more quickly postpartum.

That is why it is crucial during labor to have confidence in your ability to combine and coordinate muscle groups for relaxation and control. An alert woman with good abdominal muscles that she can effectively coordinate with the expulsive urge and pelvic floor release in labor can exert a considerable amount of voluntary force to speed along the second stage of delivery and to relax when necessary.

The EXERCISE PLUS Program Strengthens the Back

As we've mentioned before, backache is one of the most common complaints women have as their pregnancy progresses. You may notice that as your center of gravity shifts forward, you'll try to compensate by leaning farther back on your heels while standing. You may even slouch. This will only cause your pelvis to tilt farther forward with the additional weight, which in turn will stretch the abdominal muscles more and put additional strain on your back.

That is why it is so important to concentrate while lying or standing on keeping your pelvis tilted. The exercises in our program will help you do that. You will be pulling your pelvis upward and backward by contracting your abdominal muscles, and pushing it forward by tightening your buttocks. In other words, you will pull your pelvis up in front with your abdominal muscles, and down in back with your buttock muscles. This is precisely the action described in The Pelvic Tilt, Exercise 10. It is a movement that can be done when you are standing, walking, or even lying down.

In addition, our leg exercises concentrate on strengthening the thigh muscles. Strong and tight thigh muscles provide additional support for your spine.

The overall relaxation you'll feel due to breathing rhythmically during each exercise will help relax the shoulder and neck muscles, which in turn will aid in correcting any tendency to hunch or slouch forward.

The result of all this corrective movement is good posture. Students of the EXERCISE PLUS program, particularly the expectant mothers, always remark after only two or three classes that the first improvement they notice is they stand straighter and taller.

You will notice this too, for it is the first, and one of the most important, benefits of EXERCISE PLUS. Your body will immediately begin to align itself the way nature intended. You will stand, sit, and walk with proper posture, and you will adjust your body so that it can better carry your baby and yourself.

This proper body alignment takes place, quite simply, because the EXERCISE PLUS program is a method of thorough body conditioning, with special concentration on your back, stomach, buttock, and thigh muscles, all of which need to work together to help you stand straighter.

As we mentioned earlier, the exercises are based on dancers' warm-up exercises, and involve stretching and strengthening coupled with rhythmic breathing. Breathing rhythmically results in maximum benefits, as you exercise not only your musculatory but your circulatory and respiratory systems as well.

EXERCISE PLUS: *The Stretch-and-Strengthen Way to Health and Beauty*

When we say our exercises are based on dancers' warm-up exercises, we do not mean dancers' ballet routines. We are not interested in forming the bulging muscles one often sees on highly trained ballet dancers. Rather, the exercises are designed for quite the opposite result. We want to elongate your muscles by showing you how to use your own body resistance to push, tighten, and stretch them as far as you can.

This may sound strenuous at first, but in reality it should be no more of a strain than the simple stretch you probably already do in the morning upon awakening. To make sure the exercises are not too strenuous, we've designed them to be done almost entirely on a mat on the floor.

Because you do the exercises on the floor (not standing rigidly at a ballet bar), and because you will be breathing rhythmically during each routine, you should experience little or no afterpain, no stiffness even the day after your first complete workout.

To understand what these exercises accomplish, take a few seconds right now to do a simple stretch-and-strengthen exercise.

Relax as you read this paragraph, whether you are sitting or standing. Hold the book in one hand and lift the other arm straight out in front of you. Keeping your shoulders relaxed and down, reach for the wall in front of you. Reach with your fingertips as you tighten your elbow, pushing your fingers away from your body as hard as you can without moving your shoulders. Keep reaching farther and farther, tightening harder and harder, for a few more seconds. Now, relax your arm and resume whatever position you were in.

You have just done a lot of exercising. You've stretched the muscles in your upper and lower arm by elongating them. You've strengthened and firmed those muscles by contracting and tightening them very hard. We will work every part of your body in much the same way.

Always keep in mind that, as our gynecologist friend said, "the childbearing year is not a time of illness. We no longer tell women they should remain or become inactive during their pregnancy. Instead, we encourage them to begin exercising during this period, and to think of this as a lifetime pattern.

"By doing these stretch-and-strengthen exercises, coupled with rhythmic breathing, you can expect to build and maintain optimum muscle strength and length. The good nutrition habits you're going to build during these nine months will certainly be enhanced by exercises. Any tension or anxiety that creeps up on you will be relieved. And, most important, you should begin to think of these exercises as a major component of your healthy life."

Chapter 2

Your Changing Body and Image

As more and more women began signing up for the EXERCISE PLUS Program for Expectant Mothers, it became obvious that they were genuinely concerned about staying in shape while pregnant. It also became obvious that they were very concerned about their pregnant shape.

One mother-to-be, quoted in a story *The New York Times* wrote on our classes, expressed it best when she said:

> I felt myself becoming clumsy even though I knew what was happening to my body. I know there is nothing to be ashamed of, but it is very hard not to feel awkward in a regular exercise class. The pacing and breathing exercises are perfect. Olinda said we wouldn't be sore afterward, and I wasn't. I was floored. I just feel great after the classes.

Although it was a great relief for these women to be able to relax completely in a class filled with other women in their same "shape," we felt they should be equally at ease with their body image when not with a homogeneous group.

"Women react to the changes going on right before their very eyes, depending on the body image they started with," Nancy

Cuddihy told us. "We have several models in our midwifery program, women who use their bodies in their work, and some are absolutely appalled at the changes and verbalize it, yet they want to have a baby very much. On the other hand, some women who never thought of themselves as attractive at all have had a positive reaction to the changes taking place; they've decided they love their pregnant bodies. Most women have some reaction to the changes in their breasts. Large-breasted women for the most part hate the changes; they feel very heavy, sore, and tender; they hate to be touched; and they have to get two and three different-sized bras. Women who are small-breasted love it because they've blossomed.

"If a woman has had to struggle with her body image, her weight, all her life, she's probably going to be more anxious, perhaps be more ready to exercise.

"A partner's response to a pregnant woman's body is also important. What is her family telling her about how to conduct this pregnancy? Her husband may be appalled that she's out there at the gym, pregnant. Exploring all these feelings is so important."

We agreed with Nancy and hope you will want to explore your own feelings about your body as your pregnancy progresses.

It will be good to keep in mind, as one gynecologist recently pointed out to us, that "many husbands love the novelty of the changes their pregnant wives go through, particularly increased breast size. Also, the rounding out of the angles of their bodies is attractive to most men. Many even find women far more sexually desirable in early pregnancy than in nonpregnancy."

This same doctor also stressed that if both partners are assured there is no possibility of harming the pregnancy, normal sexual relations can continue.

"If the woman feels she is desired and wanted, if her man makes her feel desirable and wanted, this makes all the difference," he said.

"It is during the second trimester—a transition period for a woman—when her attitude about herself, her third trimester, and her delivery will be molded. She has the true evidence that she is pregnant: Her abdomen is enlarged, breathing is not yet difficult, and she can feel the baby move. Her abdomen is still not sufficiently enlarged, however, to interfere with coitus, which indeed should be encouraged. If sexuality is preserved during this period, if her husband makes her feel desirable and in no sense grotesque, she will enter her third trimester with fluidity and ease, and won't even notice the transition. Coitus can continue into the third trimester.

"It is the last trimester when a woman will be the recipient of the rewards for having exercised and maintained a positive body image throughout the earlier stages of her pregnancy. She'll have less lower back pain, less cramping, and in general will feel a great deal better about herself. The fact that she only has a little bit more of the pregnancy to go also helps."

Theodora (Teddy) Grauer, a mother of three and a registered nurse with an M.S. degree, has been teaching childbirth preparation classes for the last eight years, and also teaches nursing at Adelphi University in Garden City, New York. For the last two years she has been regularly taking the EXERCISE PLUS classes herself. "As soon as I began taking Lazar's classes, I incorporated his breathing techniques, as well as many of his exercises, into the Lamaze exercise classes that I teach. I had heard so much about Lazar's classes, and it was all true—they make me feel simply wonderful. My students respond in the same way.

"I find among my students that while some don't like the changes they undergo during pregnancy, many just love being pregnant. There are those who first discover their bodies when they become pregnant. It is the first time they really touch, feel, and look at themselves. For most, it is a state of almost being 'superhealthy,' and they truly enjoy it. Doing regular exercises enhances these good feelings they have about themselves.

"The very nature of the exercises at EXERCISE PLUS is that they can make anybody feel terrific about herself. You can do them at your own pace, it's just you and your body. You feel better because you've attacked specific problem areas in pregnancy —the pelvic tilt does wonders for lower backache. The tightening and relaxing of the pelvic floor muscles is a great aid in delivery.

"Being in touch with your body enhances your feeling about being in control, which in turn enhances how you feel about yourself. Feeling good about yourself can't help but improve how you feel about the way you look as well."

During the childbearing year developments take place in two areas simultaneously. While you yourself are undergoing physical and emotional changes, the fetus is growing and developing a life of its own. The development of the fetus may sometimes make you feel out of control because in a very real sense, much of what is happening on this level *is* out of your control.

That is why this is a particularly good time for you to understand not only what is happening to your own body, but also what happens during the growth of the child inside you. While knowing what is happening inside your body will not let you be in any more control of these changes, this knowledge will certainly help you deal with the changes in a less mystified and much more relaxed manner.

An average pregnancy will last around forty weeks, and can be broken up into three trimesters, or three 3-month periods.

The First Trimester

Physically the first clue you will probably have that you are pregnant is a missed period. And there might be some vaginal spotting when the implantation of the fertilized egg occurs between five and a half and seven days after conception.

We'd like to suggest that you see a doctor as early in your pregnancy as possible for a complete physical checkup. Your doctor will be able to tell as early as three weeks after conception if you are pregnant, and can usually confirm this six weeks after your last period. The doctor will give you a pelvic exam, during which he or she will be looking for changes in the color and tone of your cervix and uterus.

But besides a pelvic exam, it is wise at this time to have a general overall exam and provide your doctor with a complete medical history. Bring along any records you may have, and fill the doctor in on any previous pregnancies and your menstrual history.

Make a mental note, or take a list along, to make sure none of the following is skipped: breast exam and Pap smear; urinalysis; weight and blood pressure; blood tests for type and Rh factor, as well as anemia; rubella check; and blood sugar test. Also, discuss with the doctor the need for supplemental vitamins and minerals, especially iron and calcium.

After this first complete examination, the doctor will probably want to see you monthly until your eighth month, when he or she will see you twice. In your ninth month, you'll see the doctor weekly to check the baby's heartbeat and the opening and thinning of your cervix.

Once you have discovered you are pregnant, you may notice some of the following fairly common physical changes, although they should not be too intense.

You may have increased urination, due to increased hormonal changes. The pituitary hormones affect the adrenal glands, which change the water balance in your body, and you retain more body water. Also, your growing uterus is already beginning to press against your bladder.

Because a rise in progesterone levels also relaxes the smooth muscles in the digestive tract, your bowel movements may become irregular. The increased pressure of the uterus on the intestines, and a decrease in your activities—if you are tired and resting more —may cause constipation.

There might be an increase in vaginal secretions, since the amount and chemical makeup of the vaginal fluids are also changing.

Your breasts will probably swell and may even throb and hurt, and your milk glands will begin to develop. Veins may become more prominent with the increased bood supply to the breasts. Your nipples and the area around them, the areola, may darken and become broader.

Nausea, either mild or enough to cause you to vomit, is a common complaint during this period. This is due to the increase in estrogen, which can cause irritation in the stomach.

No matter how mild, when you are nauseated you really don't feel like doing anything physical. At the same time, you want to remain active. To get the nausea under control as much as possible, here are some helpful hints: Instead of big meals, eat lightly frequently. Avoid greasy, spicy foods, and don't fast. Try munching on dry toast or crackers shortly after getting up in the morning. Check with your doctor or midwife for some other helpful aids.

In about your tenth or eleventh week of pregnancy, your pelvic bones begin to separate as the joints between the bones widen and become movable. Sometimes this can cause the separating bones to come together and pinch the sciatic nerve, which you will feel in your buttocks and down the backs of your legs.

During these first three months you may have mixed feelings about being pregnant and becoming a mother. Your emotions may range from joy to depression, from feelings of completion to ones of isolation and anxiety. Zillions of questions will pop into your head, which is perhaps one of the reasons you've gotten this book.

Becoming knowledgeable about what is happening to you will be a great help in dealing with these unexpected emotional changes. Beginning your EXERCISE PLUS program early in your pregnancy can also help alleviate a good deal of the anxiety and depression you may go through and make you feel more in control of your emotions.

Although you will notice your own physical and emotional changes during the first trimester, the growth of the embryo as it becomes a fetus takes place without your feeling much of what is happening because everything is on such a minute scale. But it is such a fantastic process, we'll go into it briefly here so that you can know what is going on at each stage as your baby grows.

Within the first month, the embryo, which is about the size of a small white kidney bean, has millions of cells that have already developed to carry out specific functions, and a primitive heart has formed. The embryo is embedded in the uterus and is drawing nutrition from it.

By the end of the eighth week, the initial formation of the organs is complete, and the embryo becomes a complete, though miniscule, human being weighing about one ounce. Sex is apparent, a skeleton of cartilage is growing, and the first bone cells have appeared. The embryo is now referred to as a fetus.

The placenta, umbilical cord, and amniotic sac (bag of waters) are developing and functioning as a support system for the fetus.

Second Trimester

It is the growth of the amniotic sac, which gradually enlarges the uterus and in turn the abdomen, that causes the overt sign of pregnancy. This becomes outwardly obvious in about your fourth month. Your waist is becoming thicker; your clothes are tight. Your womb is beginning to swell below your waist and you'll feel light movements of the fetus.

Now is also the time you begin to gain weight. A thoroughly nutritious but careful calorie-wise diet must be adhered to. Too much weight gain at any stage will only add to your discomfort, and make movement and exercise more difficult.

Many of the circulatory changes that began during your first trimester continue throughout your second. Blood volume continues to increase as your bone marrow produces more blood corpuscles and as you drink and retain more fluid. During this period you will definitely need more iron. Even your heart is changing position and increasing slightly in size. You may salivate and sweat more.

Outwardly your skin may darken—around the nipples and in a line from the navel to the pubic area. Sometimes the pigment in your face darkens, forming a kind of mask, which will go away after birth.

On awakening your legs and feet may cramp. Exercise is particularly beneficial during this period if for no other reason than it helps the circulatory system, and aids in keeping you warm.

The skin on your breasts and abdomen may become dry when it begins to stretch, often causing lines called "stretch marks." Keep these two areas moist and supple by bathing with your favorite oil and massaging the skin with additional oil.

Since your breasts are beginning to feel heavier, it is a good idea to wear a support bra now. Although you still have no milk, you may notice a thin secretion from your breasts.

Your bowels and digestive system may function even slower now than during the first trimester. The result, unless you continue to concentrate on a good diet, can be indigestion, constipation, and heartburn. To help relieve these discomforts eat small portions, avoid spicy foods like pizza, drink lots of fluids, concentrate on whole grains (especially whole-wheat bread) and on fresh fruits and vegetables, and continue your regular exercise program.

Veins and blood vessels, because of pressure from the pelvic organs, may not be functioning as well. This can cause hemorrhoids, varicose veins, and perhaps even nosebleeds.

Again, exercise will help the blood flow through your body, alleviating some of these discomforts. Just the mere fact that you will be lifting your legs and feet off the floor during exercise reduces some of this buildup of pressure.

Naturally, as a concerned expectant mother, you will want to stop or cut down on smoking. Many studies have shown a higher number of premature births among smoking mothers. It is also best not to drink as much coffee, to drink only a small amount of alcohol, and to rest as much as you can.

During this second trimester your emotions will be trying to catch up to the physical changes and adjust to them. You may want to take some time now for introspection.

How do you feel about your new shape? How do your man and your family feel about you? Are you getting the right answers to your many questions? Intercourse during pregnancy is almost always harmless, but often depends on individual physical facts and feelings. Have you discussed the subject with your doctor and explored these feelings with your man to your satisfaction? Examining these feelings and knowing about the changes you are undergoing will help to make childbearing much more relaxed and enjoyable.

During the second trimester the fetus measures between seven and eleven inches and grows in weight from one to three pounds. As we've said, this is the time you begin to feel the fetus's movements (called "quickening"), and the doctor will be able to hear its heartbeat.

Your baby's bones are growing, its arm and leg joints and teeth are starting to form. As fat is deposited under the skin, the fetus becomes smoother, rounder, and less wrinkled and red. Muscular reflexes are developing at the eyelids, palms, and feet. Swallowing reflexes start, and thumbsucking takes place. Premature births of around twenty-four weeks can often survive in intensive care units.

Third Trimester

You are now nearing the end of your pregnancy. Your uterus is large and hard to the touch, and you can feel your baby. It moves around a lot now, and will be lying in its own particular position.

Because of pressure on the bladder, you may feel a need to urinate even when you can't. Lying on your stomach is increasingly uncomfortable. Shortness of breath may occur, since the uterus is even causing pressure on the lungs, and your diaphragm may be moved up as much as in inch.

You are still gaining weight, and indigestion is still common, since your uterus is pushing the stomach up and even flattening it. To alleviate discomfort from indigestion, drink lots of liquids, eat bland foods such as toast, cooked whole-grain cereal, soft-boiled eggs, milk and mashed potatoes. You can then add broiled meat or fish, but chew very well. Try relaxing your abdomen and the muscles around your stomach. Avoid excessive consumption of alcohol or eating spicy foods.

Your navel protrudes, and you walk differently. You may find you are leaning back even farther to balance the increased weight in front, which can cause backaches. This discomfort can be eased greatly, of course, by exercising.

The pelvic joints are much more separated. When the baby's head settles into your pelvis (called "dropping" or "lightening") a good deal of the pressure comes off the stomach, and you may even feel lighter.

Swelling ankles are common now because the average woman can retain from six to thirteen pints of liquid, half of this amount in the last ten weeks before delivery.

Your baby is maturing rapidly, gaining weight and strength. By the time it is ready to be born, all the organs will have increased their weight 120 times since they were first formed at two months. The baby's weight will have increased five billion times since fertilization, and its length, twelve and a half times from crown to heel! Growth slows down just before delivery, then there is a rapid speeding up the first few days after birth.

In general, it isn't until the eighth month that your extra weight and heaviness become truly bothersome. By this time you will probably look and feel bulky. Some women think of themselves as enormous. It is extremely difficult for them to get comfortable toward the end of their pregnancy, and many can't even bend over to put on their shoes. Most comment on this time as being marked by feelings of just waiting.

By doing the exercises in this book, you will be able to reduce many discomforts, aches, and pains. You will also have more confidence in your body's ability to function properly for a safe delivery.

Teddy Grauer pointed out to us how much the EXERCISE PLUS program is a help, particularly in the third trimester, in feeling and looking better.

"Women who have difficulty sleeping in the third trimester can get even more mileage out of these exercises if they'll repeat a few before going to sleep," she says. "Just doing the rhythmic breathing and head rolls while in bed will help you sleep better. Having learned how to use your body helps in placing it more comfortably in bed. You've gotten in touch with your body and learned to have control over how you feel.

"These exercises really do tone, stretch, and strengthen your entire body, and increase the blood flow. You've used muscles that most modern women don't ever use, and you will need to use during delivery."

A doctor friend of ours, one of the leading gyneocolgists at New York's Mt. Sinai Hospital, observed, "It's really in the third trimester when you'll benefit most from having exercised. It's in this last period when the postural changes and limitation of deep breathing, which may well have been absent in midtrimester, will become troublesome. If you've done these exercises, they will have been prophylactic, so you won't even realize the benefits because you won't suffer anywhere near what you would if you had not exercised."

The doctor went on to talk about the positive physical and emotional benefits our exercises have during labor.

"Labor is quite a physical feat," he emphasizes. "If you have exercised, you'll be able to push more forcefully and for longer periods of time—you're in better physical shape. Increased or enhanced breathing ability helps tremendously.

"If you've been practicing relaxation throughout your pregnancy, it is worth a great deal. Commonly our control of body muscles is very limited. Our ability to isolate various groups of muscles is at times very difficult. The simplest way to get someone to relax muscles is to tighten them first, which I've observed you do repeatedly in the EXERCISE PLUS program.

"One of the big problems with pushing in the second stage of labor, if you do not have total control, is that you must differentiate between two actions: tightening rectal or abdominal musculature and, by the same token, relaxing perineal musculature.

"Many women act in totally the opposite way. They will tighten abdominal musculature and tighten perineal musculature in a single unit, ending up trying to push a baby through a space that has been contracted simultaneously. This increases trauma, decreases progress in terms of descent, and not uncommonly necessitates forceps delivery."

Other doctors have also told us of this problem. When they ask patients to relax the perineal muscle, some are unable to do so without simultaneously relaxing abdominal muscles. This means they have eliminated force, which pushes the baby down. It is an all-or-nothing principle. Either their entire body becomes tense, or it relaxes totally. It is this lack of coordination, or inability to isolate several different muscle systems so that they can do different things simultaneously, that is the difficulty.

"Also, in an era when many women are having their first child, they don't know whether they're going to be able to go all the way through labor or not," the doctor went on to point out. "They will end up with an epidural anesthesia. This is not unlike a spinal, except the local anesthetic never enters the spinal cord, so the patient is able to control her musculature but is not able to feel. This can be very difficult because there is no sensory knowledge of what is going on."

It is in this realm that it is most important for a woman to become so familiar with voluntarily controlling these muscle groups that she will be able to do so even in the absence of sensory feedback. If you have the ability to both push and simultaneously relax the muscles you can't feel, progress will still be excellent and painless even if you have no sensory feedback.

Other women (because they have no sensory feedback and are relatively unfamiliar with how to mentally control these muscle groups) become totally uncoordinated and unable to push. The end result, as mentioned before, is that without sensory feedback, they can't control the muscles, and forceps delivery is absolutely necessary.

The doctor was quick to emphasize that forceps delivery under these circumstances poses no problem. It becomes a fast delivery and a safe delivery. But it is disappointing to the woman. "She may feel she didn't succeed all the way, that she got up to ninety-nine and three quarters percent there, and just couldn't make it the last inch of the way," he said.

In the last ten years about 98 percent of this doctor's patients have gone through either natural or prepared childbirth. Those situations which require general anesthesia—totally knocking a patient out—for simple vaginal delivery have virtually disappeared. He only administers general anesthesia for occasional emergencies, such as a breech position, a difficult forceps delivery, or fetal distress, where rapid delivery must be accomplished. He no longer induces labor either, and finds this to be true of other doctors pretty much everywhere.

"There is little doubt that more and more pregnant women are exercising, and of course this is terrific," he told us. "As I've said, there is a great feeling of accomplishment when you've achieved any goal you've set for yourself. Being able to go all the way with your delivery is a tremendous feeling."

We asked him about husbands and their role in pregnancy and delivery. "In my practice I'd say that about ninety-five percent of the husbands are present during labor and delivery," he told us.

"Since so many husbands are now so involved, I'd like to suggest that you encourage the women who use your book to have their husbands read the exercises to them while they do them. They can make their exercise hour a team effort. This is great conditioning for actual labor. It is never too soon to learn to respond to the voice of your man, since he will be the one to guide you through labor."

Most women have come to realize that nature doesn't simply whisper into their ears the things they need to know about pregnancy and motherhood. Fears can develop on many levels, and reducing those fears can be accomplished more by a genuine effort to learn about and prepare for a child's birth than by pure instinct.

It is good to remember again at this time that you do have control over your own very personal childbearing experience, and that 95 percent of all deliveries are normal.

In fact, you should be feeling very good about yourself. You have already planned to start an exercise program that is tailored specifically to your needs as an expectant mother. This fact puts you in control, and you are in control because, quite simply, you care about how you feel and how you look.

You don't have to be a bionic woman or an athlete to go through pregnancy or childbirth. On the other hand, you don't want to be underexercised because of any superstitions or unknown fears you may have about exercising during pregnancy.

(There are still some women who believe that if they raise their arms above their heads while pregnant, the umbilical cord may wrap around the baby's head and choke it!)

Consult your doctor if you have any misgivings about exercising. If your pre-pregnancy medical history or pregnancy itself is unusual, or if you experience any discomfort while exercising, then be sure to work closely with the doctor before starting or continuing your exercise routines. But if you lead a normal, fairly active life, see your doctor regularly, secure permission to exercise, then begin the EXERCISE PLUS program today.

As Nancy Cuddihy said after observing Olinda's class, "If you've never done a stitch of exercise, find out you're pregnant—you could do these exercises with safety and with reassurance you're not going to do your body or your baby any harm. There is that degree of safety in the EXERCISE PLUS program."

Chapter 3

The EXERCISE PLUS
Program for Expectant Mothers:
The Exercises

Since trained supervision is not always available, we've tried in this book to help you understand the principles of the exercises and how the body functions as you perform them, so that you can be your own guide. Be sure to modify any routine to your own needs: what your prior training or lack is; what stage of pregnancy you are in; and how much tolerance you have. We've designed each exercise carefully, and we've provided you with the desired number of repetitions. Before you begin, though, we'd like to suggest how we feel you should proceed.

Start out by reading through all the exercises in this chapter, one at a time, visualizing yourself going through each of the movements.

Read through each exercise a second and a third time, studying how one movement flows into the other, how the first warm-up exercises prepare you for the more strenuous ones, then how the final exercises reinforce the ones preceding, aligning your body for perfect balance and control.

When you're ready to begin, select the most appropriate spot in your home for your workout. We recommend that you choose a comfortable, quiet, and spacious area covered by a rug, an exercise mat, or an old blanket you don't mind placing on the floor. Wear a leotard, gym shorts (or underwear and a T-shirt), loose and comfortable clothes, or nothing at all—whatever you feel you can move most easily in.

In our studio we never use music while exercising because we feel you should find your own natural body rhythm to move to; we suggest you do yours in quiet at home also. You might want to take the phone off the hook, subdue the lighting, and right from the start think of this time and space as your exercise domain. Setting aside the same two to three hours a week, each and every week, will help reinforce this period as a time you regularly commit to improving your body from head to toe.

Start your exercise regime slowly. Begin with the first five exercises, mastering each individual position before moving on to the next. Repeat these five for a couple of days until you know them by heart and can move from one to the other in one continuous movement.

Then add on Exercises 6 through 11 for several days until again you can move through the first eleven without interruption. The next sequence should include Exercises 12 through 20. Then do the last five, the only ones done while standing.

In a short time you will have gradually learned all twenty-five exercises by heart, and you'll be moving easily from one to another. Your ultimate goal is to do them without pausing from one movement to another—as though all twenty-five together make up one continuous exercise. Remember, always do them in the sequence we've presented them—each movement builds on the one preceding and prepares you for the one to follow.

If you are doing the exercises alone, it's always a good idea to read through them each time before starting, in order to reinforce proper positioning and sequence even after you've learned them by heart. Keep the book close by for easy referral.

If your husband or a friend is going to participate with you by reading the exercises out loud, be sure to communicate the tempo you're most comfortable with, and try and maintain that rhythm from one movement to another.

This should be the beginning, then, for you of what we hope will become a lifetime habit of the EXERCISE PLUS program. As we've said earlier, you are strongly motivated right now because you want to maximize your health and strength during pregnancy for a better labor and delivery. These twenty-five exercises, plus proper nutrition, rest, and doctor's care, are going to get you in wonderful shape for the big event.

Just as important will be the exercise regime you set up for yourself after delivery and continually thereafter. Once you see how good you're going to look and feel, we're sure you'll want to continue your EXERCISE PLUS exercises, to stay in such terrific shape.

Start today. They are as easy as turning the page.

The EXERCISE PLUS Exercises

1. The Neck and Spine Stretch: In Two Parts
2. Rhythmic Breathing
3. The Roll Up
4. Foot Exercises: In Two Parts
    Part 1: Flex and Point
    Part 2: Foot Circles
5. The Pendulum
6. The Side Bend, One Leg Bent
7. Side and Forward Bends, Open Legs
8. Forward Stretch Sitting, One Bent Leg
9. Forward Stretch Sitting, Both Legs Straight
10. The Pelvic Tilt
11. The Long Stretch
12. The Inner Thigh Stretch
13. Sitting Leg Lifts, for Front of Thigh
14. Sitting Leg Lifts, for Inner Thigh
15. Lying-down Leg Lifts, for Side of Upper Thigh
16. Lying-down Leg Lifts, for Inner Thigh
17. The Pelvic Stretch
18. The Press
19. The Bird
20. Neck Stretches
21. The Standing Side Bend
22. The Standing Windmill
23. The Standing Forward Bend
24. The Back of Thigh Stretch
25. Relaxation

Three Postpartum Exercises

10A. The Rollback and Sit-up Return
11A. Long Pelvic Tilt, on the Stomach
16A. The Ring, on the Stomach

1. THE NECK AND SPINE STRETCH: IN TWO PARTS
This exercise releases tension in the neck, shoulder area, and upper back. It also tightens the stomach muscles, as do all the exercises in the program.

Sit up tall on the mat, legs crossed Indian style, back very straight. Remember to relax your shoulders completely (concentrate on pressing your shoulders down into your armpits). When you exhale, pull in your stomach as much as you can to protect the spine. The abdominal contraction will be the major force in successfully bringing your head forward and down, stretching and rounding the back. Place your hands on the back of your head, not on your neck.

Part One
1. Sitting tall, clasp your hands behind your head. Elbows to the back wall, lift your chin up. Inhale on 2 counts.

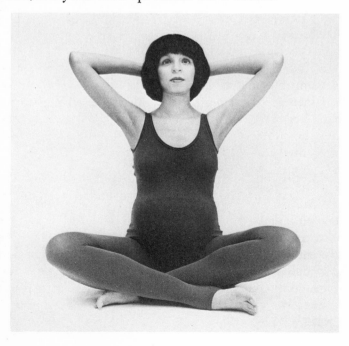

2. As you exhale, drop your chin on your chest and pull in your stomach. Drop your elbows and stretch your neck and spine, rounding your back completely. Relax your shoulders.

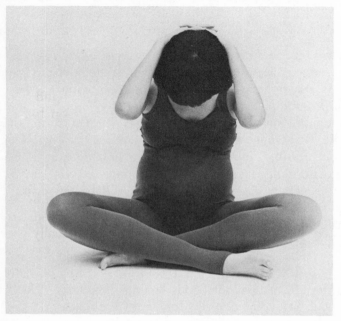

3. Inhale as you return to a sit-up, rolling up your spine, bringing your elbows way back and your chin up.

Repeat 4 times.

The fourth time you stretch forward, as in step 2, hold this position for more stretch farther down your spine, all the way to the lower back.

Part Two

1. Inhale deeply on 2 counts, relaxing your body but keeping your head down and your back in the rounded position.

2. Exhale, pulling in your stomach until you feel it is touching your spine. Tighten your buttocks at the same time. This will tilt the pelvis farther back and help the abdominal muscles to contract even more. Pull your head down gently, bringing it as far forward as you can, your chin into your chest. The idea is to round the back completely, stretching the spine all the way down to the lower back.

Repeat inhaling and exhaling 4 times, maintaining the rounded position.

After the fourth inhale and exhale, slowly roll up your spine, vertebra by vertebra, pushing your head down toward your stomach, as if uncurling. Relax your shoulders and drop your arms by your sides.

2. RHYTHMIC BREATHING

Deep rhythmic breathing increases lung capacity and relaxes you. It will be used throughout the book in preparation for each exercise.

The technique used in rhythmic breathing—filling your body with air as you inhale, emptying and flattening it as you exhale—is the correct way to breathe at all times. If it is not already your normal breathing pattern, it should become so from here on.

Lie down on your back. Bend your legs with your ankles and knees slightly apart. Relax your entire body, especially your shoulders. Keep the back of your neck long against the mat, your chin toward your chest (you should be able to see the entire wall in front of you). Place your hands on your stomach. This is your basic breathing position.

1. Inhale evenly and deeply on 4 counts. As you breathe in, fill your torso completely with air from the pubic bone upward through your chest (as though you were a balloon).

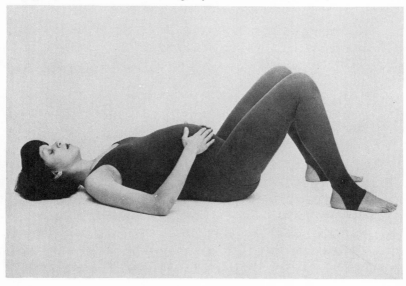

2. Exhale slowly and evenly, emptying your torso completely by contracting your abdomen, shrinking your chest, waistline, and abdomen against your spine, and flattening your spine completely against the mat. Remember to keep your shoulders relaxed and your neck long against the mat.

Repeat 6 times, each time breathing in and out rhythmically.

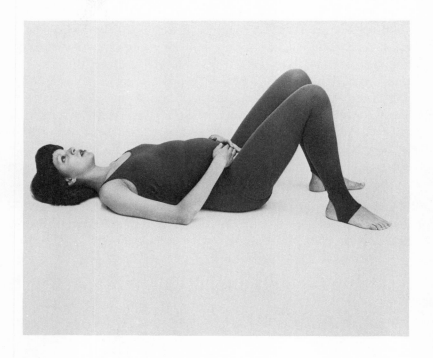

3. THE ROLL UP

This exercise is excellent for toning and tightening the abdominal muscles, which are the major muscles used to lift the head and shoulders off the floor.

Remain lying on your back. Keep both legs bent, your ankles and knees slightly apart. Place both hands under your head.

1. Inhale deeply on 2 counts.

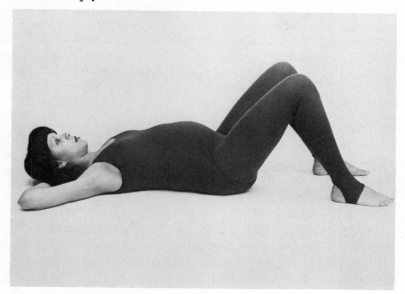

2. As you exhale, pull in your stomach, bring your elbows together, and slowly lift your head and shoulders off the floor. Tighten your buttocks as much as you can as you come up, and contract your abdomen against your spine, harder and harder. Keep your neck and shoulders relaxed. Remember, it is the ab-

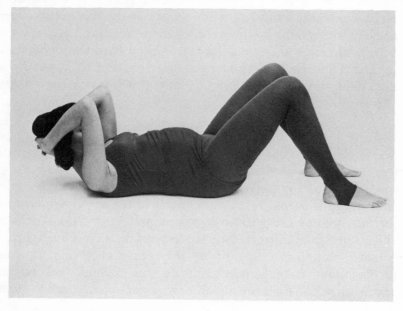

dominal muscles that are working here to lift your head and shoulders off the floor, not the neck and shoulder muscles.

3. Inhale on 2 counts. Exhale as you slowly roll back to the mat, vertebra by vertebra, keeping your abdomen contracted all the way down, your shoulders and neck relaxed.

Repeat 4 times.

Each time come up a little higher as though trying to sit up. Relax your neck and shoulders completely as you come up and roll back to the mat. Keep your feet on the floor.
    Relax, stretch out both legs long, and shake them gently.

4. FOOT EXERCISES: IN TWO PARTS
Foot exercises are a particularly good preparation for labor and delivery. The flexing of the legs and feet stretches and strengthens every muscle in the ankles, arches, shins, calves, and thighs. The flexibility you get from holding your legs in this position stretches the hip joints wide. Your arms are being exercised and strengthened at the same time as your legs. The tremendous increase in blood flow warms up the legs and feet as well as the whole body, and helps prevent varicose veins.
    Because the feet are so often underexercised, you may feel cramping in the toes and arches. If so, just rest your feet a moment, then continue; the cramping will go away as the feet get stronger. The shins are another underexercised area. You may feel a burning sensation since these muscles are worked hard throughout the exercises. This can be slightly uncomfortable, but it's a good sign you're doing the exercises correctly; it too will lessen as your feet and legs get stronger.

Part One: Flex and Point
Place both knees on your chest, separating them. Hold your knees and try to pull them toward your armpits. Lift your elbows up off the floor and keep them up throughout the exercise (this action strengthens and tones the muscles in the upper arms). Flex your feet, toes pointing toward your shins.
    There are four distinct foot movements in Part One: curling the toes, pointing the toes, lifting the toes, and flexing the feet. The first two accompany the inhale; the second two accompany the exhale. You'll breathe in as you curl your toes and point

them; breathe out as you lift your toes and flex your feet. The harder you can execute all four movements, the more beneficial. The smoother the actions, the better. Coordinating the movements with the breathing may be confusing at first, but you will soon acquire the rhythm of the exercise.

Starting with flexed feet, inhale on 2 counts as you . . .

1. Curl your toes absolutely tight, making fists with them. Then . . .

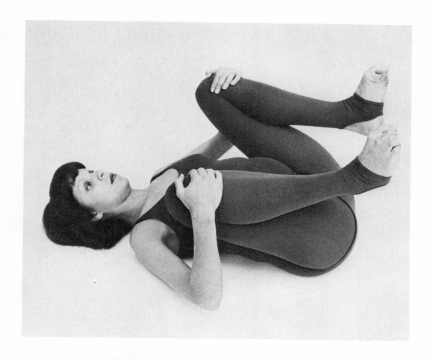

2. Keeping your toes curled, point your feet downward, and point your toes hard. Include your big and little toes in all these movements. With your feet pointed down, exhale on 2 counts as you . . .

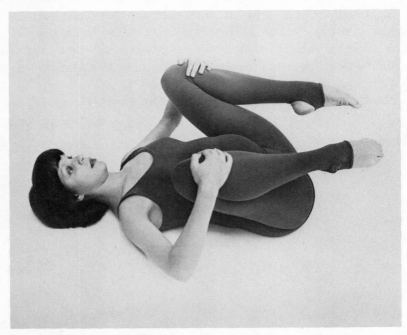

3. Lift your toes up and back as hard as you can. It helps to separate the toes while in this position. Keeping the toes lifted and spread . . .

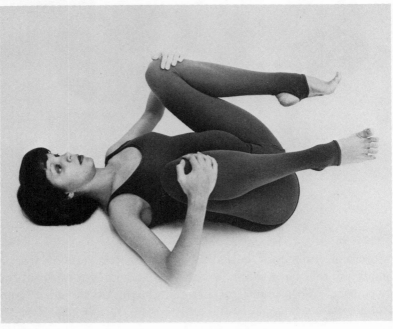

4. Lift your feet up and way back, flexing them as hard as you can, toes still spread.

Repeat this exercise 6 times.

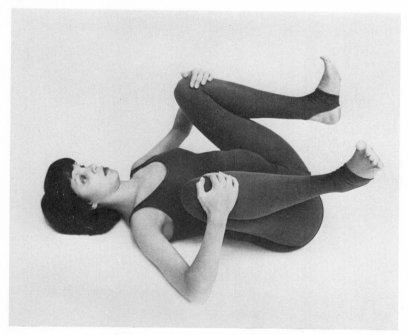

The rhythm you will want to maintain throughout depends on co-ordinating the breathing and the foot movements. Remember: Inhale, curl your toes, and point your toes. Exhale, lift your toes up, and flex your feet. With your feet still flexed after the sixth set of exercises, prepare for Part Two.

Part Two: Foot Circles

Remain in the same position as in Part One. Concentrate on keeping your legs pulled way back, knees toward the armpits. There should be very little movement of the leg as the feet circle; the steadier the legs remain, the more the muscles will be exercised. Remember to keep your elbows up throughout the exercise in order to work your arms.

The foot circles are really one continuous movement in two directions. First, you will circle both feet inward, downward, outward, and upward 6 times. Then, you will reverse the motion, circling outward, downward, inward, and upward 6 times.

Starting where you ended Part One, with both feet flexed way back, inhale on 2 counts as you . . .

1. Curl your toes and turn them inward toward each other (pigeon-toed), moving them in a circular motion inward and downward until you're pointing your toes hard, then continuing . . .

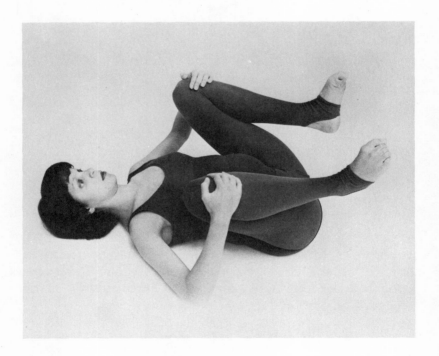

Exhale on 2 counts as you . . .

2. Circle your feet outward, away from each other, spreading your toes wide and bringing your feet way back to a flexed position, where you are ready to begin again.

Repeat 6 times, circling your feet inward each time.

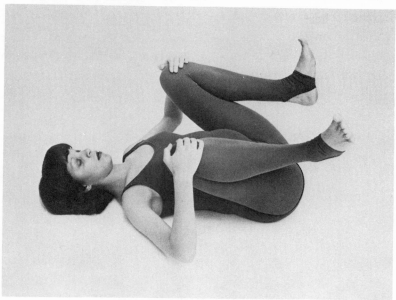

On completion of the sixth circle, with feet flexed, reverse the circle. As you inhale on 2 counts . . .

1. Curl your toes and turn your feet outward, away from each other, moving in a continuous motion outward until you are pointing your toes hard, then continuing . . .

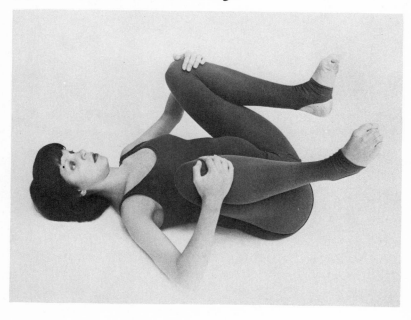

Exhale on 2 counts as you . . .

2. Circle your feet inward, toward each other (pigeon-toed) with toes spread wide, and bring your feet back to a flexed position, where you are ready to begin again.

Repeat 6 times, circling your feet outward each time.

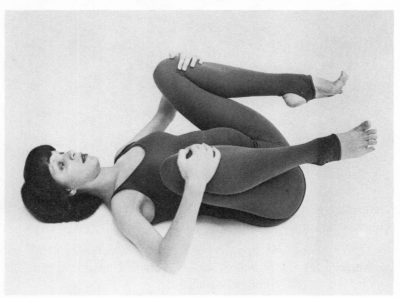

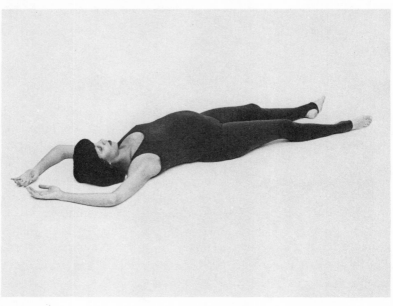

Relax your body completely by stretching out your arms and legs, shaking them loose, and taking a few deep breaths.

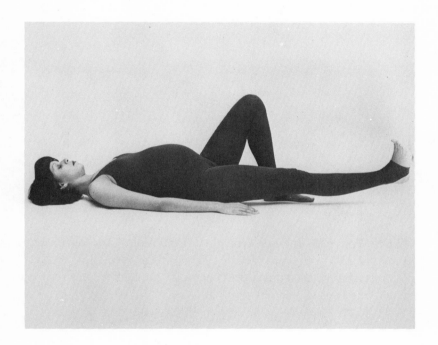

5. THE PENDULUM

This exercise is especially good for the stomach, since you are using your abdominal muscles to keep your back flat against the mat as you lift and lower your leg. It also strengthens the thigh muscles, tightens the buttocks, stretches the muscles in the back of the leg, and strengthens the lower back area.

Lie flat on your back, arms by your sides, neck long, and shoulders relaxed. Bend one leg enough to keep your spine against the mat; turn the foot in slightly. Stretch the other leg long and flex the foot. Remember as you exhale to contract the abdominal muscles completely: These muscles are the ones that are primarily responsible for lifting and lowering the leg.

1. Inhale on 2 counts.

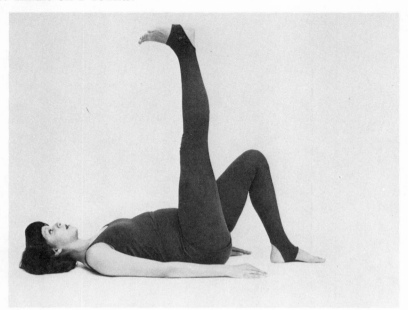

2. Exhale and pull in your stomach, tightening your buttocks, as you slowly lift your extended leg straight up into the air. Reach for the ceiling with your heel, keeping your knee straight, and flexing your foot as hard as you can.

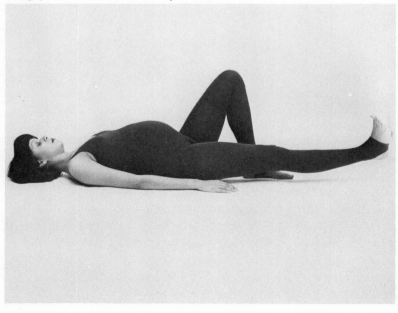

3. Inhale on 2 counts as you hold your leg in the air.

4. Exhale as you slowly lower your leg but don't let the heel touch the ground. While you're lowering the leg, tighten your buttocks, flatten your stomach completely, and keep reaching for the front wall with your heel, tightening your knee and flexing your foot as hard as you can. Keep your shoulders relaxed, your neck long, and your chin on your chest, and keep pressing the small of your back into the mat, using your tightened abdominal muscles. Remember, don't touch down with this leg.

Repeat 4 times with the right leg. Repeat 4 times with the left leg.

Relax on the mat, shaking out both legs.

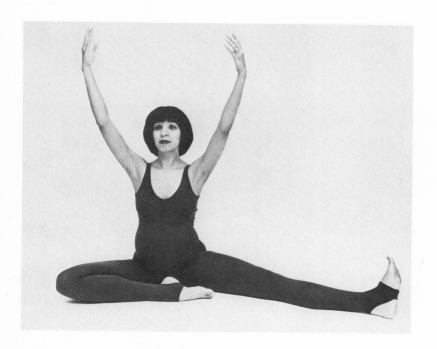

6. The Side Bend, One Leg Bent

This exercise stretches the muscles along your sides and in your arms. It also increases the stretch in the inner thigh and firms up the muscles in the upper thigh.

Sit up straight and tall. Bend one leg. Extend the other leg to the side as far as you can. Straighten and stretch this leg long, pressing the knee into the mat. Flex your foot and try to lift your heel off the floor. Try not to let the heel touch the floor through-out the exercise. Lift both arms way up into the air, but keep your shoulders down and relaxed.

1. Inhale on 2 counts, reaching for the ceiling with both arms long, elbows straight.

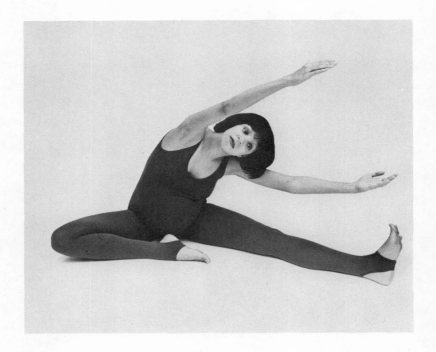

2. As you exhale, flatten your stomach, tighten your buttocks, and bend to the side. Drop your head as though trying to put your ear on your extended leg. Go easy. Stretch both arms long, reaching way past your foot, with your heel off the floor.

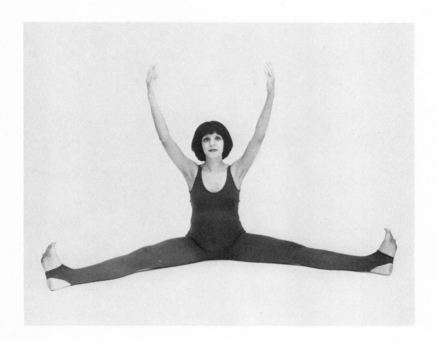

3. Inhale as you come up, reaching for the ceiling with your fingertips.

Repeat 4 times to the right. Repeat 4 times to the left.

7. SIDE AND FORWARD BENDS, OPEN LEGS

Side Bend, Open Legs

This is an extension of Exercise 6. It increases and intensifies the stretch in the sides, arms, and inner thighs, and it trims the waistline.

Sit up straight and tall, stretching both legs to the side, opening them as wide as you can. Remember, as you inhale and come up, lift your arms way up into the air, stretch them long and feel your elbows tighten, and reach with your fingertips for the ceiling. Keep both legs long, feet flexed, knees pressed into the mat. Try to lift both heels off the floor and keep them lifted, even as you bend to both sides.

1. Inhale on 2 counts, reaching for the ceiling with both arms long, elbows straight.

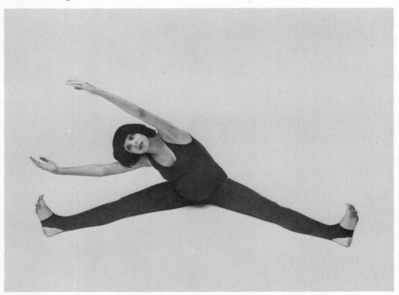

2. As you exhale, flatten your stomach, tighten your buttocks, and bend to the right side. Drop your head as though trying to put your ear on your right leg. Go easy. Stretch both arms long, reaching way past the right foot, both heels off the floor.

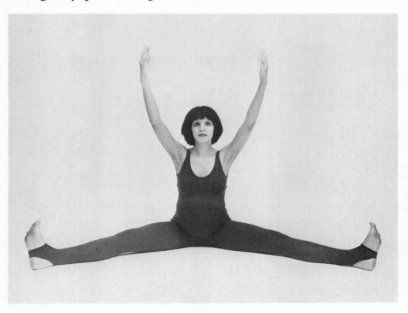

3. Inhale as you come up, reaching for the ceiling with your fingertips.

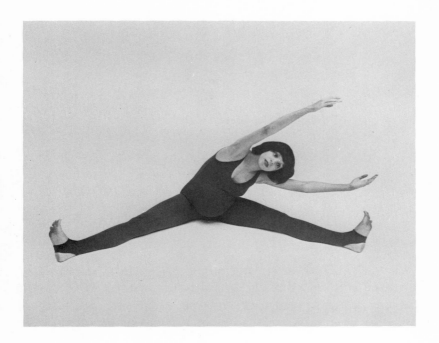

4. Exhale, flatten your stomach, tighten your buttocks, and bend to the left side. Drop your head as though trying to put your ear on your left leg. Go easy. Stretch both arms long, reaching way past your left foot, both heels off the floor.

5. Inhale as you come up, reaching for the ceiling with your fingertips.

Repeat the side bends 8 times, alternating to the right and to the left, 4 times on each side.

After the eighth bend, as you come up tall, prepare to bend forward. The forward bend will increase both the stretch in the spine and the stretch and flexibility in the hips and inner thighs.

Forward Bend, Open Legs
1. Inhale on 2 counts, reaching for the ceiling with your fingertips, back straight, sitting slightly forward on your hips.

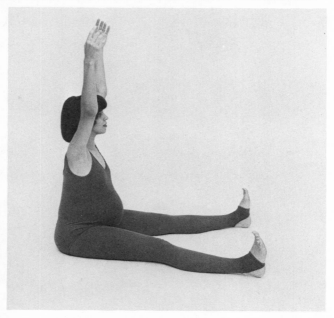

2. As you exhale, flatten your stomach, tighten your buttocks, drop your chin on your chest, and bend forward. Stretch your arms long and reach for the front wall. Make sure you relax the muscles in your neck and shoulders. Keep your legs long, knees pressed into the mat, both feet flexed, and heels off the floor.

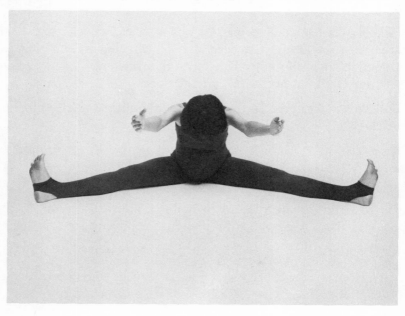

3. Inhale as you come up, reaching for the ceiling with both arms long and elbows straight, stretching your body long and sitting slightly forward on your hips, back straight.

Repeat the forward bend 4 times.

Close your legs and shake them out. Shake out both arms and relax for a moment.

8. Forward Stretch Sitting, One Leg Bent

This exercise fully stretches the hamstrings and the spine, and it firms the muscles in the thighs and calves.

Sit up tall with one leg bent, one leg straight out in front of you. To really work each leg, flex your foot back completely. Press your knee down against the mat until you feel your upper thigh muscle tighten completely and your heel comes up off the floor. Stretch your leg long, away from the hip, as though trying to touch the front wall with your heel.

1. Inhale deeply, lifting your arms way up into the air, reaching for the ceiling with your fingertips. Try to put your arms, fully stretched, way behind your ears.

2. As you exhale, relax your shoulders, pull in your stomach, drop your head on your chest and gently bend forward, reaching for the front wall way past your toes. Remember, try to keep your heel off the floor as you bend forward, flexing your foot way back.

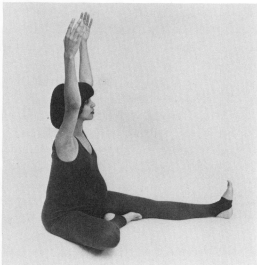

3. Inhale and come up, arms way behind your ears, back straight and body long.

Repeat 4 times with your right leg stretched way out front.
Repeat 4 times with your left leg stretched way out front.

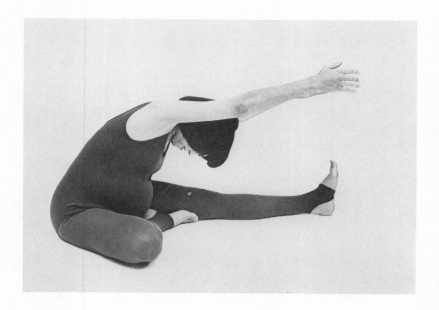

Each time you bend forward, try to reach a little farther. But remember, how far forward you can bend will depend on how big your stomach is! As your pregnancy progresses, shift your abdomen slightly away from your outstretched leg to increase the bend.

(Caution: If you feel any lower back pain during this exercise, bend the knee of the outstretched leg slightly.)

After you come up from the fourth forward stretch over your left leg, prepare for the next exercise by stretching both legs straight out in front of you, far enough apart to accommodate your stomach.

9. FORWARD STRETCH SITTING, BOTH LEGS STRAIGHT

This exercise is especially good for stretching the muscles in the backs of the legs—a great warm-up exercise for any sport, even walking.

Sit up straight with both legs stretched in front of you, slightly apart, feet flexed, arms way up into the air. Check yourself in this starting position by making sure that your shoulders are down, and that your arms are straight and long and way behind your ears. Straighten your legs out long and tighten them by pressing your thighs and knees into the mat and flexing both feet so that the heels come off the floor.

1. Inhale on 2 counts, reaching taller and taller. Tighten your buttocks completely, gripping the mat with buttocks and thighs.

2. Exhale, flattening your stomach against your spine to protect it as you bend forward in one long, slow, sweeping motion and reach way past your toes. Go easy and let your head drop on your chest so that your neck muscles are not tense.

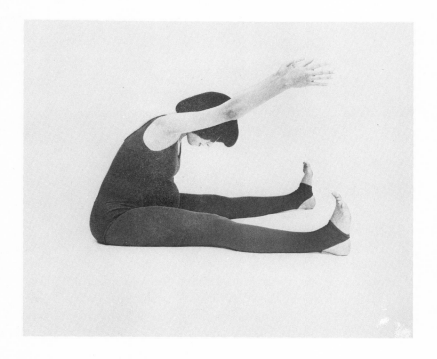

3. Inhale as you come up, keeping your arms and legs long and straight, feet flexed, arms way behind your ears.

Repeat forward stretch 4 times.

(Remember, if your lower back bothers you, bend both knees slightly as you stretch forward.)

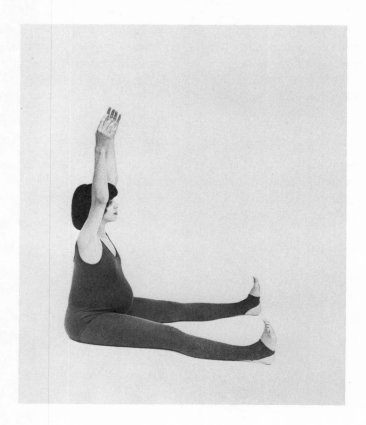

10. THE PELVIC TILT

This exercise is very important during pregnancy (and post-partum) because it corrects the body's tendency to move forward off-center as it begins to compensate for the expanding uterus. The Pelvic Tilt aligns the body, improves the posture, and relieves lower backache and stiffness. It strengthens the abdominal muscles and tightens the buttocks. It also tightens and strengthens the muscles in the thighs, groin, and pelvic floor.

Lie down on the mat in your basic breathing position, your arms by your sides, your knees bent, your ankles together, and your feet pointed straight toward the front wall.

1. Inhale on 2 counts, filling your torso with air from abdomen to chest as in the rhythmic breathing exercise. Keep your neck and shoulders relaxed, your chin down.

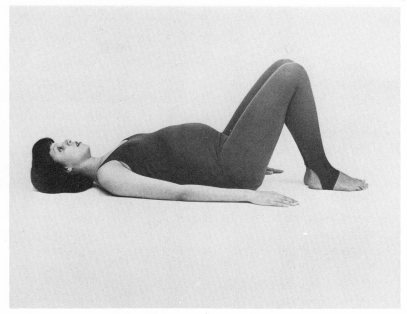

2. As you exhale, flatten your stomach, tighten your buttocks, squeeze your thighs together, and tilt your pelvis, curling it upward and toward your waist. Just lift your tailbone slightly off the floor, but keep your waistline on the mat.

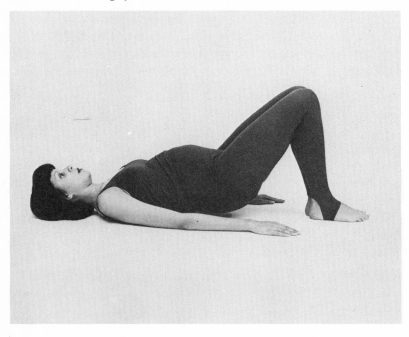

3. As you inhale, relax back onto the mat, vertebra by vertebra.
Repeat 6 times.

For more of a workout, the sixth time you tilt your pelvis, hold this position and inhale deeply on 2 counts. Don't touch down with your tailbone as you let all the air out, pull in your stomach completely and shrink at your waistline. Tighten your buttocks as much as you can, squeezing and tightening your thighs until you feel a burning sensation.

Repeat the breathing 4 times, keeping your tailbone off the floor and your waistline on the mat each time you breathe in and out.

After the fourth time, inhale as you relax slowly back onto the mat, rolling down your spine, vertebra by vertebra, with your hips being the last to touch down. Shake out your legs.

11. THE LONG STRETCH
This stretch is excellent for body alignment and posture. It is also extremely relaxing and sure to become a favorite.

Lying on the mat, stretch your legs long and point your toes. Stretch your arms over your head. Keep your chin on your chest, your shoulders and neck relaxed, and your eyes looking at the wall in front of you.

The object is to flatten the entire spine against the mat, from the back of your neck to the tip of your tailbone. This is not easy to do and will take some practice. Each time you do the exercise, concentrate harder and harder on pressing your spine into the mat.

1. Inhale on 2 counts, your arms and legs relaxed.

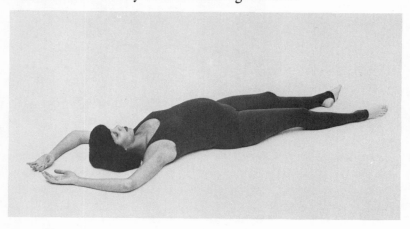

2. As you exhale, pull in your stomach and press your waistline into the mat. Stretch your body long as you reach for the back wall with your fingertips and the front wall with your toes. Do not tense your neck and shoulders—stretch your arms out but keep your shoulders well down as if you're trying to press them into your armpits.

Relax as you inhale.

Repeat 6 times.

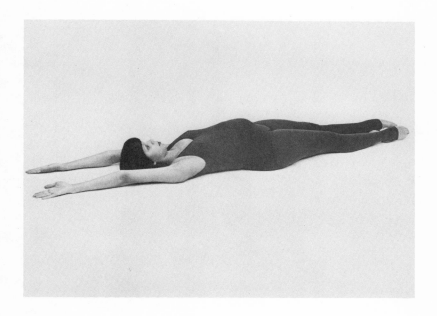

Remember, each time you exhale, stretch your body longer and longer. Reach harder and harder for the front and back walls as if you were trying to touch them with your fingers and toes. Shrink in at your waist and chest as you squeeze in your stomach to press your waist into the mat.

Eventually, as your abdominal muscles get stronger and your spine more supple, you will be able to tighten your stomach completely and press your entire spine into the mat.

Shake out your arms and legs.

12. THE INNER THIGH STRETCH

This exercise is especially good for stretching and firming up the inner thigh muscles, and for strengthening the lower back.

It is important to make sure your whole back remains on the mat at all times during the exercise. Make certain that both hips don't move, and do not let your lower back arch.

Lie on the mat, knees bent and slightly apart, your arms by your sides. Keep your chin on your chest, your shoulders and neck relaxed.

1. As you inhale on 2 counts, bend one leg to your chest, flexing the foot.

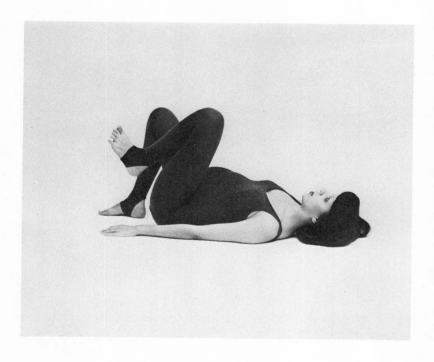

2. As you exhale, pull in your stomach and extend your leg straight up into the air, reaching for the ceiling with your heel. With your leg in the air, inhale on 2 counts.

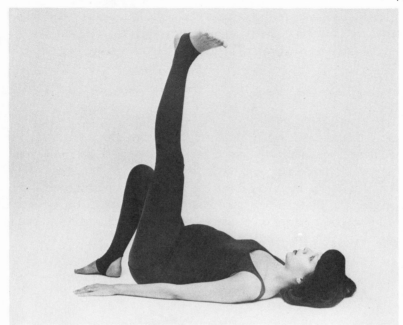

3. Exhale and slowly open the straight leg to the side, at the same time opening the bent leg to the other side. Keeping both legs open wide, inhale on 2 counts.

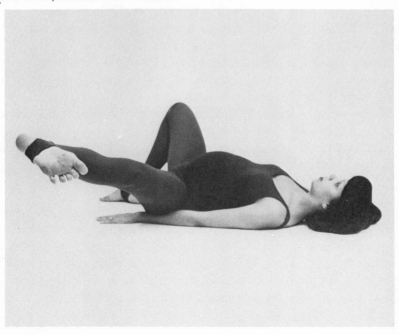

4. As you exhale, pull in your stomach and bring your legs together. Slowly raise the straight leg up into the air and bring the bent leg back to the center. Bend the straight leg to your chest.

Repeat 4 times with the right leg. Repeat 4 times with the left leg.

Remember, as you open the straight leg to the side, keep your foot flexed hard and your knee pressed in tight. Each time you do this, try to move the outstretched leg closer to your ear. At the same time, press open the bent leg as much as possible, pushing it closer to the floor. This positioning makes it easier on your back and helps you control the outstretched leg better. It also helps keep your hips stable and your back from arching.

13. SITTING LEG LIFTS, FOR FRONT OF THIGH
In this exercise you are not only strengthening the muscles in the upper thigh, you are stretching them long as well. And at the same time you are strengthening the back, particularly the lower region.

The object is to try and raise your leg off the floor without leaning back. You won't be able to lift the leg very high, but that's okay. What counts is the action of trying to lift your leg, stretching it long without leaning back. A helpful hint: To keep from leaning back, concentrate throughout on sitting forward from your hip joints with a perfectly straight back.

Sit up straight and tall, and lean slightly forward. Bend one leg and hold the ankle with both hands to brace yourself. Stretch the other leg straight out in front of you. Flex the outstretched foot, and don't touch down with your heel once you've begun.

1. Inhale on 2 counts. As you exhale, pull in your stomach against your spine as much as you can and slowly lift the outstretched leg up, lengthening it as you lift, and reach for the front wall with the foot flexed. (Note: When you lift your leg up, don't just lift it, otherwise the muscles in your upper thigh will bunch up. Instead, try to stretch your leg long, then lift it with a greater stretch each time.)

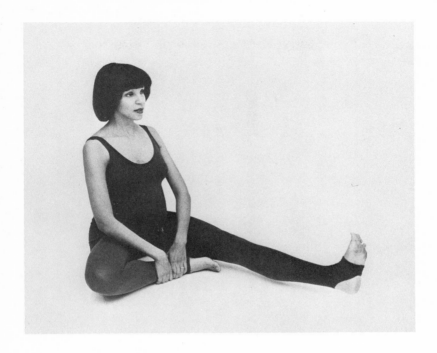

2. Inhale and lower your leg, stretching it even longer, keeping your foot flexed. Don't touch down with your heel.

Repeat 4 times with the right leg. Repeat 4 times with the left leg.

Rest, shaking out both legs.

14. SITTING LEG LIFTS, FOR INNER THIGH

This exercise is basically the same as Exercise 13, only the foot is flexed *outward*, stretching and firming the inner thigh. This routine works the back muscles as well.

Again, the object is to try and lift your leg, using a lengthening motion away from the hip joint without leaning back. If your leg comes off the floor only slightly, that's fine. Don't lean back; instead, lean slightly forward throughout the exercise. Lean from your hip joints, keeping your spin perfectly straight.

Sit up straight and tall. Bend one leg and hold the ankle with both hands to brace yourself. Stretch the other leg straight out in front of you, flexing the foot hard. Turn the flexed foot outward. Try to rotate the entire leg as much as possible, as if trying to touch the floor with your toes and point your heel toward the ceiling.

1. Inhale on 2 counts. As you exhale, pull in your stomach against your spine and slowly lift your leg, lengthening it as you lift, trying to point your heel toward the ceiling and your toes toward the floor.

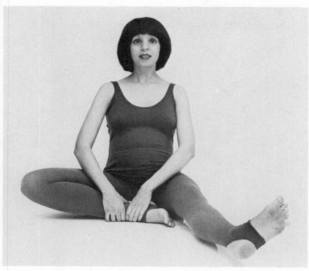

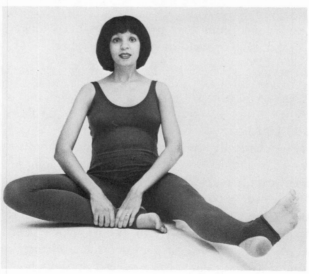

2. Inhale and lower your leg, lengthening it even more, heel still reaching for the ceiling. Don't touch down.

Repeat 4 times with the right leg. Repeat 4 times with the left leg.

Relax and rest, shaking out both legs, rounding your back slightly.

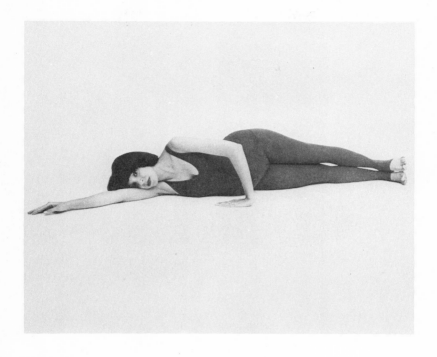

15. LYING-DOWN LEG LIFTS, FOR SIDE OF UPPER THIGHS

This is an excellent exercise for toning and reducing the outer and upper thigh; it also firms and trims the buttocks, and it tightens the abdomen.

Lie down on your side. Straighten both legs out long, one on top of the other. Put the underneath arm flat on the floor in line with your body. Use the other hand for leverage—place it in front of your chest with the elbow up. Flex both feet. As you raise and lower the top leg, your foot remains flexed and your heel is pointed toward the ceiling. When you lower the leg, don't touch down.

Remember, you don't have to lift your leg too high. The object is to keep it long so that you are stretching the outer thigh muscle as you tighten it. Trying to go too high could result in a bunching up at the waistline—do not involve the waistline in this exercise. Contracted abdominal, buttock, and thigh muscles are the only ones used in raising and lowering the leg.

1. With both knees straight, feet flexed, inhale on 2 counts.

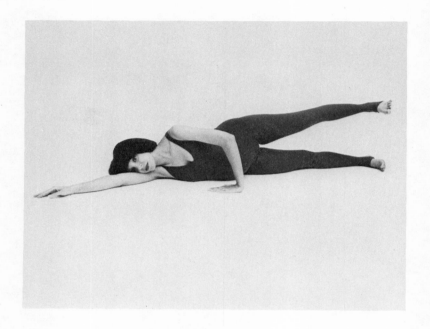

2. As you exhale on 2 counts, slowly raise the top leg, pulling in your stomach to support the movement and to prevent your back from arching. Turn your heel up to the ceiling, stretch your leg long, reaching with your foot for the front wall.

3. Inhale as you lower your leg, keeping the knee straight, the leg long, and both feet flexed. Don't touch down.

Repeat 4 times with the right leg. Repeat 4 times with the left leg.

A good way to check that you are keeping the top leg as long as possible is to make sure that both knees stay aligned throughout the exercise.

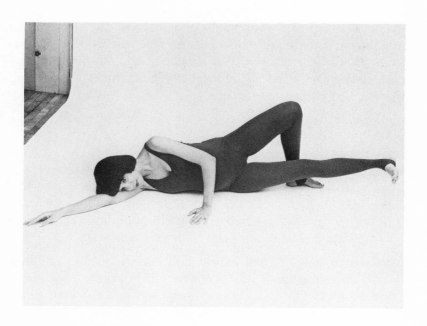

16. LYING-DOWN LEG LIFTS, FOR INNER THIGH

This variation on lying-down leg lifts concentrates on toning and trimming the inner thigh muscles.

Lie down on your side as in Exercise 15, only this time bend the top leg, with your knee facing the ceiling, and your foot on the floor in back of the bottom leg.

The object this time is to lift the bottom leg as high as you can, concentrating on squeezing your thighs together, tightening your buttocks and abdominal muscles, and tucking in your pelvis. The leg remains long, the knee straight, the foot flexed. As you slowly raise and lower your leg, try to point your heel to the ceiling. Don't touch down.

1. Inhale on 2 counts. As you exhale, pull in your stomach. Squeeze your thighs and buttocks tight, tuck your pelvis under, and lift your leg, reaching for the ceiling with your heel.

2. Exhale as you lower your leg. Don't touch down.

Repeat 4 times.

3. On the fourth lift, hold your leg in the air. Inhale on 2 counts. As you exhale, squeeze your thighs and buttocks together, flatten your stomach, straighten your knee, and flex your foot as hard as you can. Hold this position as you breathe in and out 4 times, each time increasing the stretching and tightening actions, always trying to lift your heel higher and higher.

Repeat 4 times with the right leg. Repeat 4 times with the left leg.

17. THE PELVIC STRETCH

This exercise is great for stretching the hip joints completely, the area you want to have well stretched and supple for ease in delivery.

Sit up straight. Bend your legs and bring your feet together, the soles of the feet touching. Grab your ankles with both hands—you are going to press your thighs open with your elbows.

1. Inhale on 2 counts. As you exhale, pull your stomach in and lean forward. Drop your head, relax your shoulders, round your spine, and press your thighs open. Stretch your hip joints—try to touch the mat with your thighs.

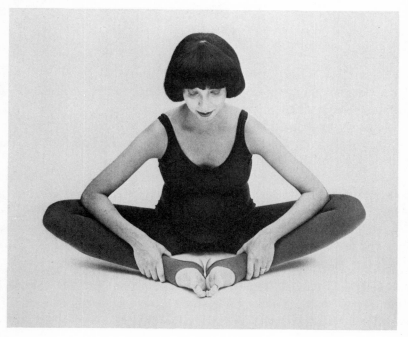

2. Relax as you inhale and come up slowly, vertebra by vertebra.

Repeat 6 times, each time pressing your thighs farther open, stretching your hip joints and pelvic area more and more.

Relax and shake out your legs.

18. The Press

This exercise is good for strengthening the arms, especially the hard-to-firm-up muscles in the upper arm near the armpits. It also firms up the chest muscles.

Sit up, legs crossed Indian style. Put your palms together in front of your chest, with your elbows up.

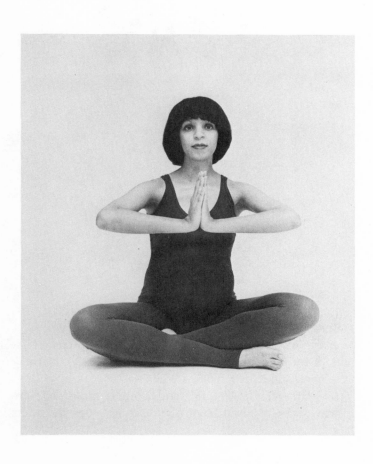

1. Inhale on 2 counts. As you exhale, press your palms tight, flatten your stomach, and slowly—keeping this pressure—lift your arms up and up. Try not to tense your shoulders; keep them down. Try to press your thighs open as you lift your arms higher and higher.

2. Inhale as you lower your arms, keeping an even pressure as you bring your hands back in front of your chest. Keep your elbows up, your knees pressed to the floor, and your back straight. Exhale.

Repeat 6 times.

Shake out your arms and relax.

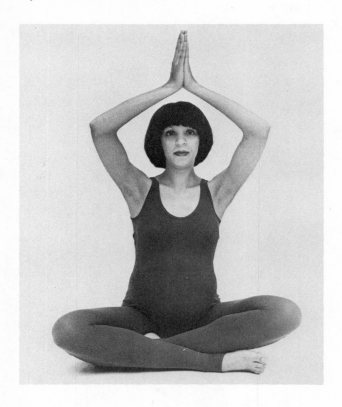

19. The Bird

This exercise is wonderful for the posture. It straightens and relaxes the shoulders by expanding and firming the muscles in the chest. It firms the neck and upper arms as well.

Still sitting up straight and tall and keeping your legs crossed, lift your arms straight out in front of you, with your shoulders well down.

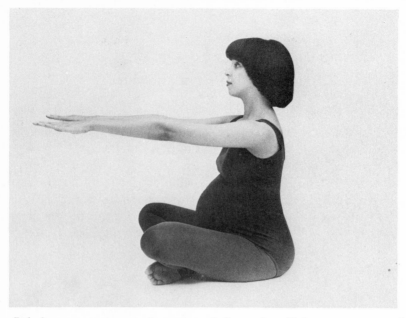

1. Inhale on 2 counts. As you exhale and pull in your stomach, slowly open your arms (like a bird) and reach for the back wall with your fingertips. Slowly lift your chin up and stretch your neck long as you reach and stretch your arms farther and farther back, keeping them long and lifting them slightly as you reach.

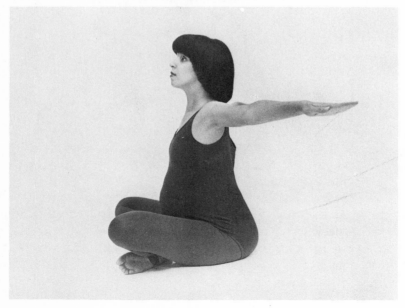

2. Inhale as you bring your arms back in front of you. Relax your shoulders and neck.

Repeat 6 times.

Take a deep breath, shake out your arms, and relax.

20. Neck Stretches

This is a terrific exercise for relaxing you all over, for strengthening the spine, and for firming the muscles in the neck.

Still sitting up tall with your legs crossed, drop your head on your chest. Make sure that both shoulders are absolutely down and that your back is straight. You will circle your neck, but instead of just going around and around, concentrate on getting the most pull and stretch out of your neck muscles as possible.

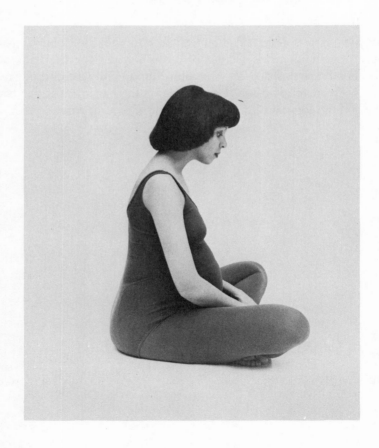

1. Inhale on 2 counts and drop your chin on your chest. As you exhale, pull in your stomach and circle your head to the right, trying to put your right ear on your right shoulder. Feel the muscles in the left side of your neck stretching long. At the same time, try to press your left shoulder down, and check that your right shoulder is also down.

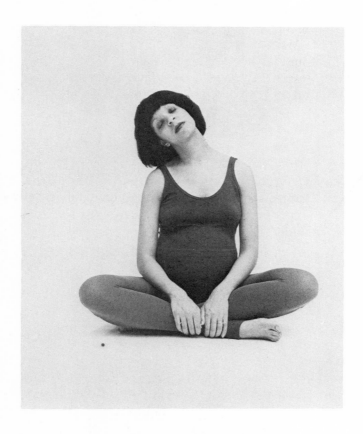

2. Inhale and continue the circle, moving your head toward the back wall. Exhale and reach with your chin for the ceiling. Your chest is lifting up as you try to look at the back wall and stretch the front of the neck long. Check that both shoulders are down, your stomach in and your back straight.

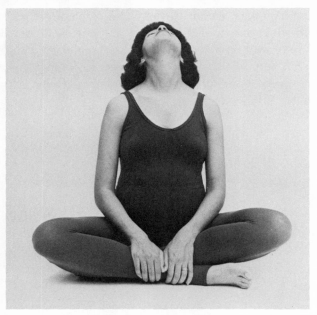

3. Inhale. As you exhale, circle your head to the left, trying to put your left ear on your left shoulder. Press your right shoulder down for a long stretch on the right side of your neck; check that your left shoulder is also down.

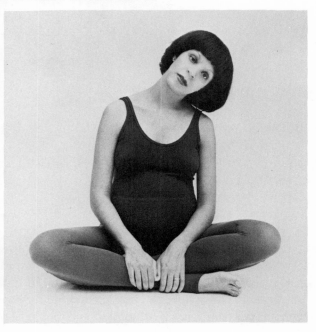

4. Inhale. Exhale as you continue the circle and stretch your head forward and down in front. Stretch the muscles in the back of your neck long as if somebody were taking you by the face and pulling your head forward and down. Keep your spine straight and long. Inhale as you lift your head up.

Repeat 4 times to the right. Repeat 4 times to the left.

Relax your back and just rest a moment.

21. THE STANDING SIDE BEND

This exercise stretches and tones the sides, trims the waistline, and firms the upper arms.

Stand up straight and tall. Separate your legs slightly and tighten them completely by pressing your knees back. Lean slightly forward on the balls of your feet. Tilt your pelvis by contracting your abdomen and tightening your buttocks and thighs. Lift your arms way up into the air, keep your shoulders relaxed.

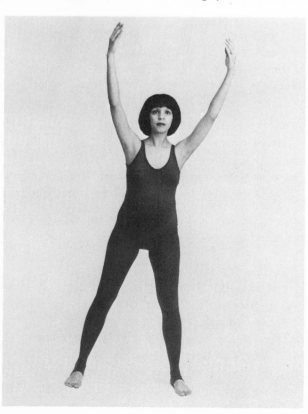

1. Inhale on 2 counts. As you exhale, pull in your stomach tight against your spine and bend at the waist to the right side as much as possible. Keep both shoulders and hips facing the front wall. Try not to let your hips move or swing.

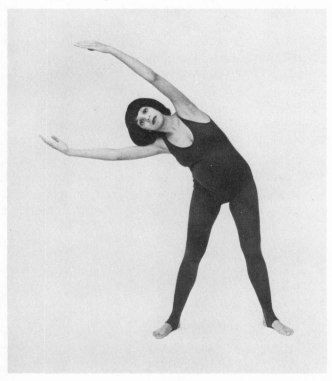

2. Inhale as you come up, reaching for the ceiling with your fingertips. Feel your elbows connected to your fingertips.

Repeat the bends 8 times, alternating to the right and to the left, 4 times on each side.

22. THE STANDING WINDMILL

This exercise is a continuation of the side bend, only this time you will move your torso in a circular motion, like a windmill, to increase the stretch and to keep your spine limber.

Legs slightly apart, reach for the ceiling with your arms. Stretch your body as long as possible, reaching up with your fingers extended. Tilt your pelvis by moving your hips toward the front and tightening your buttocks and thighs. This routine should be done totally relaxed, using no force.

1. Inhale on 2 counts. As you exhale, try to pull in your stomach against your spine, and bend slowly to the right side, reaching for the wall with your fingertips. Keep your face, shoulders, and hips in the direction of the front wall. Then slowly rotate your body, bending your knees, and begin looking at the floor. Your arms will move from the side to in front of you. Lower your body even more in a smooth motion as if you are going to sweep the floor with your hands. Pause when you are bending loosely forward, knees still bent, arms and hands dangling. Relax completely.

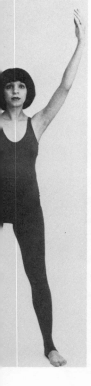
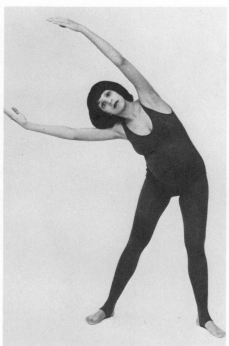
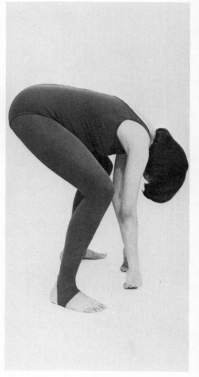

2. Inhale on 2 counts. As you exhale, slowly move to the left as though sweeping the floor, and begin reaching for the other wall with your fingertips until you are bending to the side with your shoulders, face, and hips now facing the front wall. Continue the circle as you slowly come up to a straight position. Your body should just swing as you drop down and then slowly swing as you come up—in a sweeping sort of motion.

Repeat 4 times, circling to the right. The last time, stretch your body long, standing even taller, then reverse the circle. Repeat 4 times to the left. Move right into Exercise 23.

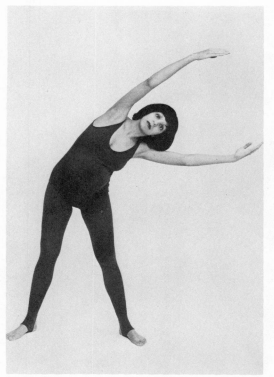 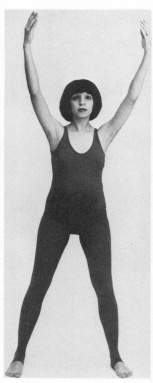

23. THE STANDING FORWARD BEND
1. Inhale on 2 counts as you come up from the last side bend.

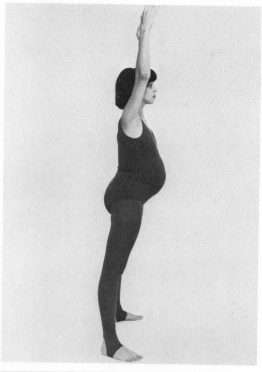

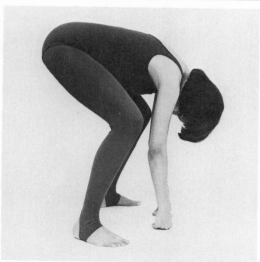

2. Exhale as you bend directly forward, bending your knees slightly. Drop your head on your chest, let your arms hang, and just collapse. Relax your shoulders; there should be no tension in your neck muscles.

3. Inhale as you come up and reach for the ceiling, stretching your body long.

Repeat 4 times. Move right into Exercise 24.

24. THE BACK OF THIGH STRETCH

1. Inhale on 2 counts as you come up from your last forward bend.

2. Exhale on 2 counts. As you bend forward this time, pull in your stomach as much as you can. Bend both knees slightly and grab the backs of your calves or ankles with both hands. Pull your head down toward your legs. Go easy as you do this—the object is to increase the stretch in the backs of the thighs.

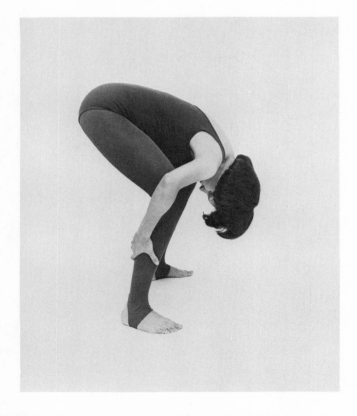

3. Inhale as you come up stretching your body long.

Repeat the stretch 4 times. Move right into Exercise 25.

25. RELAXATION

On the fourth stretch in Exercise 24, release your ankles and gently straighten your legs, letting your body hang forward loose. Shake out your head, neck, shoulders, and arms.

1. Inhale on 2 counts. Exhale as you come up slowly, vertebra by vertebra, your head down, your chin on your chest, your shoulders and arms loose and down.

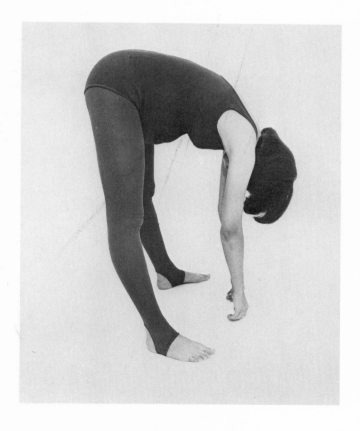

2. Inhale on 2 counts as you stand straight and tall, looking straight out in front of you, your shoulders and neck relaxed.

3. Exhale as you lift both arms slowly up into the air. Reach up with your fingertips, stretching your body long, your shoulders down and your neck relaxed, your head facing front, and your heels on the mat.

4. Inhale on 2 counts. Exhale as you open your arms wide out to the side, and slowly bring them down to your sides.

You should be standing straight and tall, your entire body in perfect alignment, relaxed, balanced, and ready for whatever your day may bring you.

Chapter 4

The EXERCISE PLUS Program for Newly Delivered Mothers: Additional Exercises

Your body has taken nine months to prepare for delivery. Fortunately, that doesn't mean it is going to take another nine months to return to your pre-pregnancy state. Immediately after delivery, your body begins its invisible process of restoration. You can aid in this restoration, and speed things up considerably, with proper exercise and diet.

It is only logical that the more fit you were before and throughout your pregnancy, the quicker you will get back into your most desired shape. As important as exercise was during pregnancy, it may be even more vital to you postpartum.

The greatest need for exercise occurs in the first week after delivery. As always, consult your doctor before beginning—especially if the birth was complicated or unusual—but, in general, it is safe to start exercising twenty-four hours after delivery, right in your hospital bed.

If you don't exercise after delivery, the muscles which have been stretched over the past nine months will remain stretched and weaken further as you resume your normal daily activities.

According to most doctors, it takes weeks for the body to readjust to the hormonal effects of pregnancy. This means that your joints and ligaments remain in their softened state for a while, and must be protected until the muscles surrounding them are restored or corrected to their former or proper length and strength. Your weakened abdominal muscles put a good deal of strain on your pelvis and lower back region. Because of the hormonal changes these areas underwent in pregnancy, they are still at risk, and care must be taken not to put undue stress on them.

By concentrating from the beginning on tightening and firming your abdominal and pelvic floor muscles, you will not only be able to protect your body, especially the lower back, from further stress, but you will be starting the important process of correcting the posture you developed, particularly in the last month of pregnancy.

Your stretched abdominal muscles, then, are going to require most of your attention postpartum. To resume a flat abdomen and good posture, with your pelvis tilted back to realign it in its correct relationship to the spine, you must concentrate on shortening and strengthening the abdominal muscles. A reminder here: Double-check with your doctor to see if you have any separation of the recti muscles—the muscles in the vertical midline of your abdomen—before beginning any abdominal exercises.

Your pelvic floor muscles also will feel slack and stretched after birth, and it is imperative that they do not remain in this state. The longer you wait to exercise your pelvic floor, the more serious the atrophy and deterioration of these muscles will be. By exercising the pelvic floor after delivery, you will be tightening these muscles to enable them to resume their role in supporting the pelvis and to reestablish sphincter control. Fortunately, the vast majority of labors and deliveries proceed smoothly. Thus, the recovery of the pelvic floor is fairly easy.

The vagina has been stretched to the extreme during delivery and the area is tender, but it has tremendous recuperative powers. As you begin tightening the pelvic floor, you may at first feel little in the vaginal region, but sensations will return quickly. If you've had stitches you may have some discomfort. Exercising this area is actually helpful in alleviating the discomfort. It is beneficial because during muscle contraction of the pelvic floor, the edges of the incision are pulled together rather than apart. There's no cause for concern, therefore, that your stitches will tear out. This gentle muscle activity also promotes healing by increasing the blood flow to the area.

You're probably going to feel pretty good postpartum, maybe even terrific. However, don't be concerned if you experience some discomforts such as sweating, loss of appetite, thirst, constipation, or increased urination as the body eliminates the accumulated fluids. Many women experience similar discomforts, but find they lessen as normal activities are resumed.

Sometimes women experience a depression or low period around three days after birth. It is best to discuss these feelings with your man and your family. If the mood swing is extreme— real highs followed by severe lows—be sure to discuss these emotional changes with your doctor. You might also discuss when you can safely resume intercourse. This should occur whenever you are fully ready, providing there are no medical constraints.

To begin getting you back in shape and to make you feel better in those first few days after birth, we've described below six exercises you can repeat as often as you want right in your hospital bed. These exercises should help alleviate any physical discomforts you may have. And, just like good exercises done any time, these six will also make you feel better about yourself emotionally. Being physically fit is the best kind of insurance for faster postpartum recovery.

With most normal deliveries, you can expect to be out of bed after twenty-four to seventy-two hours. Your own experience during labor and delivery will dictate exactly when you'll be up and about, but from the beginning while you're still in bed, you can start getting your body back into its healthy, vital state.

To avoid any strain on your backbone or any additional stretching of your abdominal muscles, we want to emphasize that you do these initial exercises in a stable position—in your bed—where support is maximal and all unnecessary effort is avoided.

The First Six Exercises: For Immediately After Birth

1. DEEP RHYTHMIC BREATHING. After the hard work you've gone through in labor and delivery, you'll need to dispel the waste products you've accumulated in your muscles and tissues, as well as the effects of any medication or anesthesia you may have received. The best way to hasten the process and to aid in resuming good blood circulation is to practice deep rhythmic breathing.

Twenty-four hours after delivery, while lying on your back in bed relaxing, take deep rhythmic breaths regularly. With your legs bent, your ankles and knees slightly apart, relax your entire body, especially your neck and shoulders. Place your hands on your stomach, and inhale evenly and deeply on 4 counts. As you inhale, fill your torso completely with air, from your pubic bone up through your chest (like a balloon). Exhale on 4 counts slowly and evenly, emptying your torso completely.

As a rule, just try for two to three deep breaths every hour or so. And always do your deep breathing whenever you do any other exercise.

This exercise will also provide intra-abdominal pressure that aids in elimination while your abdomen and pelvic floor are still in their lax state.

2. RELAX/REST/SLEEP. It is just as important to get plenty of sleep and rest and to relax fully as it is to exercise during these first few days and weeks. Remember, you've undergone terrific stress, and it takes a while for the body to heal itself after such an experience.

One of the first things you're going to want to do after delivery is to lie on your stomach. To increase the benefits of doing this, place a pillow under your hips. This will aid in relaxation, and speed up the restoration of your pelvic organs to their normal state. Lying with a pillow under your hips will also help to involute, or shrink, the uterus—that is, return it to its pre-pregnant condition and size. (Through involution the uterus automatically reduces from one-twentieth to one-twenty-fifth of its size at delivery.)

3. TIGHTEN WHOLE BODY. A good time to practice tightening the whole body is while you are lying on your stomach.

Inhale deeply on 2 counts, relaxing all over. As you exhale, pull in your abdomen, contract your buttocks and sphincter muscles, point your toes, tighten your entire leg, and tense your arms. Hold this tightened position for 4 counts, then relax your whole body as you breathe in deeply. Repeat this exercise 4 times in a row, several times during the day whenever you think of it as you lie on your stomach.

During these first few days after delivery also consciously tighten your buttocks, sphincter muscles, and pelvic floor before rising from your bed or chair. Concentrate on contracting and tightening these muscles to provide maximum support for your pelvic organs and spine every time you get up from the bed.

4. TIGHTEN PELVIC FLOOR. You can practice your Kegel exercise while you're recuperating in bed, as well as when you're urinating. Do this important exercise as often as you think of it.

While seated on the toilet, voluntarily start and then stop the urine flow several times. Let some urine out before beginning the exercise. Let a smaller amount pass each time you do the contraction.

While lying on your back relaxed, tighten the urethra in the same way you did to stop yourself from urinating. Holding the urethra tight, also tighten your vagina (you should feel this a little higher up and in the middle of your body). Continue to hold the vagina and move farther upward to tighten the muscles in the rectum. Hold for a count of 6, then release all the tension until you have relaxed to the limit. (Don't be concerned if you don't feel three distinct contractions. All the sphincter muscles seem to tighten spontaneously whenever you tighten one of them. What is important is to build up your repetitions gradually until you are doing the Kegel exercise every day, around thirty times a day.)

5. TIGHTEN ABDOMINAL MUSCLES. Initially you will want to tense, retract, and pull in your abdominal muscles to gently coax them back to their former length and strength. Don't overwork these muscles at any single time. It is better to repeat abdominal contractions a few times and frequently rather than to strain and tire them by working them too hard at one stretch. Remember, any strenuous exercise, particularly abdominal exercise, must not be attempted until there has been good recovery of the muscles in the abdominal wall and pelvic floor. How quickly you recover depends on your physical condition before and during pregnancy, and what kind of labor and delivery you've undergone.

An easy way to begin working your abdominal muscles in bed is to flatten your back against the mattress by pulling in your abdomen and slightly lifting the pelvis (this is a modification of the Pelvic Tilt exercise).

Lie on your back, bend your legs, keep your ankles together, and your arms by your sides.

Inhale deeply on 2 counts, filling your torso with air, keeping your shoulders and neck relaxed.

As you exhale, flatten your stomach, tighten your buttocks, squeeze your thighs together, and tilt your pelvis slightly, curling it upward and toward your waist. Keep your entire spine on the mattress, especially the waistline, and just lift your tailbone slightly.

Inhale and relax completely. Repeat around 4 times.

It takes about six weeks for involution of the abdominal cavity and abdominal wall. If your abdominal muscles have retained their tone, they will return to their original condition. However, as the authors of *Our Bodies, Ourselves* point out, "It is important to exercise during pregnancy and to do the exercises prescribed for the postpartum period, because the abdomen almost never comes back to its pre-pregnant condition without exercise."

6. IMPROVE CIRCULATION. You can begin immediately to improve the circulation in your legs, and tighten your stomach at the same time, by flexing and pointing your feet.

While lying relaxed on your back, straighten out both legs. Flex both feet hard and inhale deeply on 2 counts. As you exhale slowly, curl your toes down and point them hard.

Inhale as you curl your toes up and bring your feet back to the flexed position. Repeat 4 to 6 times. Perform this exercise as often as you feel comfortable doing it but don't overdo it.

Your Complete Postpartum EXERCISE PLUS Program

Once you're home and settled, you should continue daily the important six exercises we have just described whenever you're taking time out during the day to lie down and rest. They only take a little while, but will make all the difference in the world as you feel your body responding and tightening up. By the time you have your six-week checkup, your abdominal and pelvic muscles will already have improved dramatically in tone.

Around four weeks after normal delivery (six weeks after a Caesarean), you should be able to resume your twenty-five EXERCISE PLUS exercises, as well as add on the three new ones we'll describe shortly. However, if you are still passing blood, or if you begin to bleed, stop these exercises and wait until all the bleeding has ceased.

We suggest that when you resume your EXERCISE PLUS program, you go through all the exercises with as little effort as possible. In other words, for the first week simply perform each movement effortlessly, not pushing yourself to tighten or stretch any muscle too hard. Also for the first week or two, just do one half the number of repetitions you did while pregnant.

This way you will very gradually begin to recondition your entire body without putting too much strain on muscles and joints that are still in the process of recuperating. As you build your strength, increase the number of repetitions at a comfortable rate until you are doing the same number you did while pregnant.

When you go for your six-week checkup, discuss your post-partum exercise program with your doctor, and remember to ask him or her to check particularly for any abdominal muscle separation. You may even want to show your doctor this book so that he or she understands clearly just how the EXERCISE PLUS program was specifically designed for pregnant and newly delivered mothers.

In working with the women who come to our class following their delivery, we've found that by the time they're settled at home and up and about, they welcome the EXERCISE PLUS routine. In fact, most say their body craves it!

"I can't wait to get back to exercising at EXERCISE PLUS," one of our regulars recently told us. "Even though I didn't start your program until my sixth month of pregnancy, I found it enormously beneficial during labor and delivery, especially the relaxation and control it brought me with my knowledge of deep rhythmic breathing. I started immediately on your six recommended postpartum exercises while I was still in the hospital, and now I'm anxious to work out from head to toe and get back in shape."

Another client, who has been regularly attending our newly delivered mothers' exercise classes for two months, was delighted to see how her body was responding. "I was in my fourth month of pregnancy when I began EXERCISE PLUS, so I had a good five months to tone up my body. I had always thought I was in pretty good shape, but was amazed at how much stronger and firmer I was by the time I delivered than before I got pregnant! Now since I've delivered, I'm determined to look and feel even better than I did a year ago."

You'll probably also find, as you begin your EXERCISE PLUS

regime, that you're going to want to continue with it indefinitely. As your body begins to go back to its pre-pregnancy state, you, and only you, will know how satisfied you will be with that condition. If you were in excellent shape before you got pregnant, you'll of course be delighted to see your old self again. If, however, there were areas of your body you weren't exactly thrilled with, just arriving back at that state may leave you dissatisfied. With the EXERCISE PLUS program and proper eating habits, you can attain your most desired shape and stay that way (see Chapter 5 for postpartum nutrition and diet).

Three Additional Exercises

After you're doing your first twenty-five EXERCISE PLUS routines at full capacity and number of repetitions, you can add three exercises for a complete shape-up program. Practice these three new exercises the same way you did when you were learning the first exercises, until you know them by heart and can do them in one continuous movement.

Then we suggest you intersperse them throughout the first twenty-five, doing each in the following sequence:

1. The Rollback and Sit-up Return should follow Exercise 10.

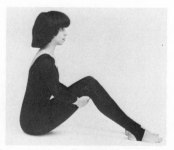

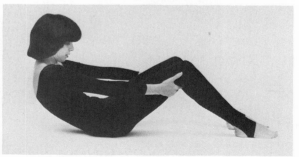

2. The Long Pelvic Tilt, on the stomach, should follow Exercise 11.

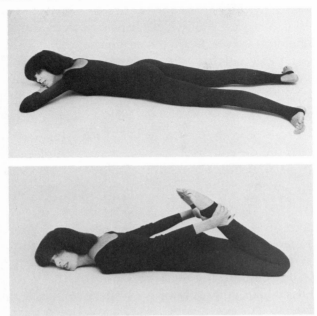

3. The Ring should follow Exercise 16.

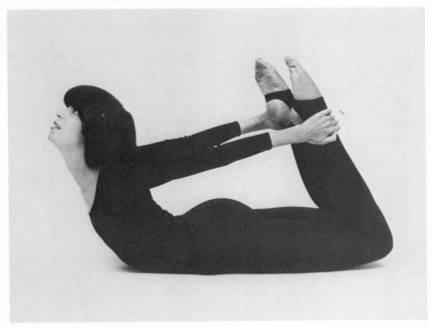

10A: The Rollback and Sit-up Return

This exercise is specifically intended to strengthen the stomach muscles. After delivery these muscles are very stretched and weak, so when you first begin this exercise, you'll need some help. Let someone hold your feet down as you do the exercise, or put them under a solid piece of furniture that will remain stable.

Sit up straight with your legs bent and slightly apart. Hold your thighs with your hands throughout the exercise.

1. Inhale on 2 counts, filling your stomach with air, and holding your spine very erect. As you exhale, drop your head on your chest and begin to roll back slowly, making sure each vertebra touches the floor, especially from the tailbone to the waistline. Go all the way down until your head is resting on the mat, with your neck long.

2. To come up, inhale deeply. As you exhale, lift your head up. Put your chin on your chest, pull your stomach muscles in as tight as possible, and then try to roll up slowly, using the contraction in your stomach muscles to come up. Put your hands on your thighs to help you up until your stomach muscles are strong enough to raise and lower your torso on their own.

Repeat 6 times.

11A: Long Pelvic Tilt, on the Stomach

This exercise will help tighten the buttocks and the backs of the thighs. You should not use the muscles in your back during this exercise, so there should be no strain on the lower back.

Lie down on your stomach, resting your head on your hands. Open and straighten your legs as much as possible, flex your feet out to the sides, and let your heels touch the floor.

1. Inhale on 2 counts. As you exhale, pull in your stomach as much as possible and squeeze your buttocks. Using a pelvic-tilt motion, try to press your pubic bone into the mat. You'll feel your buttocks tightening more and more as well as your thighs contracting.

2. Start out slowly, don't use too much force, and only hold for a second or two in the beginning. As you gain more strength in your stomach, hold for a count of 4 as you exhale, then inhale as you relax back onto the mat.

Repeat 4 times. Rest after the fourth time by totally relaxing your body on the mat for a full minute.

16A: THE RING, ON THE STOMACH

This is an excellent exercise for strengthening the back muscles, and for tightening and firming the buttocks and the backs of the thighs.

Lie down on your stomach. Bend both knees, grab your ankles, and keep your knees slightly apart. Rest your head on the floor.

1. Inhale on 2 counts in this position. As you exhale, pull in your stomach as much as possible to protect your spine. Slowly and carefully, raise your head and chest off the floor. At the same time raise your feet into the air as if trying to straighten your legs. Try to raise your thighs off the mat as well. In this position, your body looks as though it is forming a ring or circle. Go easy at first —you will feel the muscles in your back, buttocks, and the backs of your thighs contracting and tightening as you raise your body, as if you were trying to fly up into the air.

2. Inhale as you slowly let your legs down and relax back to the floor. Still holding your ankles (as in step 1), repeat the exercise very carefully at first, using no force. Gradually you can build up to straightening and tightening harder and harder.

Repeat 3 times. After the last time, rest completely by relaxing all the muscles in your body for a full minute.

This will bring your permanent set of exercises up to a total of twenty-eight. You'll find after you've done them for a while that you can go through the complete routine nonstop in forty-five minutes. As you master the entire program, you may find you'll want to increase the number of repetitions, which is fine.

Whether you reach your desired shape with the number of repetitions prescribed in the book, or whether you want to go beyond this number and repeat each exercise with greater frequency, you will be able to utilize your EXERCISE PLUS program to suit your own needs and desires. The benefits of the program, as we've said throughout the book, are quite extraordinary: relaxation, balance, control, proper body alignment, strength, flexibility, firmness, and desired shape.

You will also now have a much deeper understanding of how

your body functions at its peak. This understanding and feeling will go far to motivate you to continue a regular schedule of exercising two to three times each week. It should also provide any incentive you need to control your weight so that you do not overeat due to stress or anxiety (since you'll find you're much more relaxed). You can control your weight and at the same time eat properly by becoming aware of what goes into a good diet, and by learning the caloric and carbohydrate content of your favorite foods.

Getting in shape means you will look and feel better than you have in the past. Staying in shape means you can look and feel your best now and in the future. Proper exercise and nutrition are your best insurance for a happier, healthier, and shapelier life.

Chapter 5

The Shape You're Meant to Be In

Weight is a constant problem for a pregnant woman. It's a problem during pregnancy—the most common cause of excessive weight gain in females is pregnancy!—and after childbirth. You would be wise to talk over any weight problem you may have with your doctor before embarking on a diet. There are loads of diets on the market right now, many of which can help you take off those unwanted pounds, but you should begin one only under the advice of your physician, particularly if you are breast-feeding. He or she will guide you through your pregnancy, counseling you on how much weight to gain. Let your doctor also help you take off any weight after delivery.

According to most doctors, as United Feature Syndicate columnist Dr. Robert Newman puts it, "It is advisable for a woman to gain at least fifteen pounds during pregnancy because that amount merely represents the additional weight resulting from her developing pregnancy, the baby, amniotic fluid, extra blood, placenta, and uterus. Ideally, the average woman should actually acquire from twenty to thirty additional pounds in order to maximize fetal size and well-being."

In her excellent book *The Woman Doctor's Diet for Women*

(New York: Ballantine Books, 1979), Dr. Barbara Edelstein takes great care in pointing out the difference between a woman of normal weight who becomes pregnant and gains twenty to thirty pounds and one who is already twenty to thirty pounds overweight at the start of her pregnancy. A woman of normal weight who gains twenty-seven pounds during pregnancy can expect that up to nineteen pounds, but no more, will be lost when she delivers. These eight additional pounds are not catastrophic for a woman at her desired weight, because she can lose the excess pounds fairly easily. But a woman who is already twenty to thirty pounds overweight at the outset of pregnancy will gain at least eight pounds more. She then has an enormous amount of weight to lose after delivery to reach her desired weight.

To make matters worse, in those first six months after delivery you don't lose weight very efficiently. Your whole metabolic system has slowed down, and it takes months for it to return to what it was before pregnancy. The exception in this case is if you are breast-feeding. Here you have a golden opportunity to burn off those extra pounds fast because you're using up even more calories than you did while pregnant.

The weight you do lose during and after delivery is a combination of what the baby weighs, the contents of the uterus, and an extra five pounds of water. This amounts to losing approximately one eighth to one sixth of your body weight within just those first few days postpartum.

What your postpartum diet consists of is very important in getting your strength back, not only for yourself but for maximum health in taking care of your new baby. Plan on eating a normal, well-balanced diet. If you're nursing, you'll want to stay on the same diet you were on while pregnant, with the addition of an extra pint of milk a day. Make sure you are getting around 80 to 100 grams of protein a day.

If you're not nursing, you'll probably begin menstruating in eight weeks. If you are nursing, you ordinarily won't menstruate if your child is being *completely* breast-fed, and you probably won't ovulate. But since there is a great variation in women during this period, you should discuss birth-control methods with your doctor whether you're nursing or not. Don't rely on breast-feeding alone to provide natural contraception.

Most nutritionists seem to agree with the basis of a healthy day's diet as set down by Adelle Davis in *Let's Eat Right to Keep Fit*

(New York: Harcourt Brace Jovanovich Inc., 1970). In order to get the nutrients you need in their most concentrated forms, try to see that your daily diet consists of the following:

A quart of milk (six cups if you are nursing) in the form of whole milk, skim milk, buttermilk, yogurt, or fortified milk;

Whole-grain breads and cereals (amount depending on your weight and activity);

Vitamin A in the form of raw and cooked vegetables, liver, and butter;

Whole citrus fruits and juices, plus fruits and juices other than citrus;

Vitamin D from egg yolks, fish, and fish-liver oils;

Iodized salt (keep below five grams daily);

One to two tablespoons cold-pressed vegetable oils (again, adjust according to your weight and activity) in salad dressings, in cooking, and as seasoning (keep the oil refrigerated); and

Two servings of meat, fowl, fish, eggs, cheese, nuts, or beans.

If you are happy with the rate at which you're losing weight after delivery and find you can stay with your normal eating habits and still be your desired shape, then you are lucky indeed and need not concern yourself with dietary restrictions.

If, on the other hand, you are concerned with your excess weight and are having difficulty losing it, the following advice should prove helpful.

Learn to Count Carbohydrates as Well as Calories

The noted nutritionist and food researcher, Dr. Carlton Fredericks, is very concerned with the millions of us who are overweight. In his book *Carlton Fredericks' Calorie and Carbohydrate Guide* (New York: Pocket Books, 1977), he says that

> Excess weight, even a small amount, is a burden. Have you ever tried carrying a ten-pound package around all day? It makes your heart work harder. It puts a strain on your circulation. It helps to bring on diabetes and worse. . . . Even a few extra pounds tilt the scales away from well-being and toward a long list of common disorders. If you have the know-how to get rid of those extra pounds and then keep them off, you can do a lot for your health as well as your figure. That know-how begins with informing yourself about the calorie and carbohydrate values of everyday foods.

Dr. Fredericks' advice on counting carbohydrates as well as calories makes a lot of sense, especially for women. Dr. Edelstein discovered that calorie-counting alone is useful only as an approximate measure for the overweight female. The inefficient way her body converts food, especially carbohydrates, to energy sets her apart from men and thin women. It is still important to know the calorie content of foods, Dr. Edelstein points out, but it is even more important to keep the carbohydrate level low and the protein level high for a steadier weight loss. This means restricting your intake of carbohydrates in the form of highly refined flour and refined sugars of all kinds, including honey, molasses, etc. Complex carbohydrates such as grains, vegetables, and fruits in an unrefined, minimally processed form are necessary for a well-balanced diet, but the amount must be monitored to insure weight loss in women.

The fact of the matter is, says Dr. Edelstein,

> Women are the fatter sex. By the time we're adults, we have twice as much fat as men. We burn from 10 to 15 calories per pound of weight where men burn from 17 to 20 doing the same thing, yet our appetites are identical.

All female hormones are naturally fat-producing and fat-hoarding, which means that women convert food into fat much easier than men do. Women require fewer calories than men—two to five calories less per pound—yet often eat as much or more than men do!

Why this propensity to fat in females? Because women are designed as baby receptacles, says Dr. Edelstein. Nature has gone out of its way to make sure we will never be without fat, but will always be padded with a soft cushion of under-the-skin fat, just in case the fetus needs extra food, protection, and heat.

Once you are no longer pregnant, you do not need so much of that protective layer of fat. Since you're going to want to eat a well-balanced diet and still try to lose weight, the best thing you can do is take both Dr. Fredericks' and Dr. Edelstein's advice —cut down your calorie and carbohydrate intake in the form of fats and refined sugars and starches.

You can still eat a balanced diet and reduce the total calories and carbohydrates you consume by concentrating on getting at least half your calorie requirement in the form of protein. Protein is more satisfying because it is filling, while simple carbohydrates actually stimulate your hunger. At the same time, protein burns more efficiently and gives you a much more even blood-sugar level. This benefits the whole metabolic system, stabilizes moods, and creates sustained weight loss. Overweight females in particular handle protein more efficiently than carbohydrates.

Dr. Fredericks asserts that

> It's a fact that there are people who don't lose weight with simple calorie-restriction regimes, unless they also change the proportion of carbohydrates to proteins and fats in their diets. Translation: They lose if the reducing diet is low in starches and sugars; they don't if it isn't—even when the calorie values of the two diets are identical.

Sometimes this is because carbohydrates make you retain salt and thereby also retain water. If this is so, your weight won't go down significantly because you're just substituting water for fat in your tissues.

In addition to watching the calorie and carbohydrate intake, both Drs. Edelstein and Fredericks caution that it is just as important to spread your calories and carbohydrates out over three meals a day and not save them up for one or two. Most overweight females don't metabolize more than a certain number of calories per meal. If that number is exceeded, the excess is stored as fat.

In other words, if you are now over your desired weight, it is far more important for you to balance your intake of calories and carbohydrates over the day than skip a meal or two and consume them all in the evening. Unless that meal is under 500 calories, you're going to store the excess calories as fat.

You burn up a greater number of calories breaking down protein for use as energy in the body than you do breaking down carbohydrates. According to Dr. Edelstein, protein uses about 30 percent of its caloric value while being converted to energy, whereas carbohydrates use very few calories to produce energy. Therefore, an overweight woman can eat 30 percent more calories in the form of protein than carbohydrates or fat, and still stay within her caloric limits.

It looks like simple carbohydrates and fats are your enemy right now while you're trying so hard to lose weight and get yourself back in shape. Keeping the facts about proteins, fats, and carbohydrates in mind, it would be good to begin learning by heart the carbohydrate and calorie count in the foods you eat. Determine with your doctor what your calorie requirements per day should be, then try to balance those calories over three meals, getting as few of them as possible from starches and sugars and more of them from protein.

A simple way to figure your calorie requirements is this: Every pound on your body is equal to 3,500 calories. To lose a pound a week, you have to cut back by 3,500 calories that week, or 500 calories a day.

Decide *with your doctor* what you want your ideal weight to be. Multiply your ideal weight by twelve to get your daily calorie requirement. For example, if your ideal weight is 120 pounds, multiply by twelve to get 1,440 calories a day. In order to lose a pound a week to reach 120 pounds, subtract 500 calories from 1,440 and eat only 940 calories a day until you achieve your goal. To maintain your weight at 120 pounds, eat 1,440 calories a day. But remember, cut back that extensively only under your doctor's supervision.

Dr. Fredericks feels that

> at the beginning of the diet your objective is to keep your carbohydrate intake at about 60 grams daily. This is merely a starting point—some people lose successfully on more than 60 grams of carbohydrates; some do better if they eat even less than that.

Sixty grams, even 100 grams, as some nutritionists recommend, is not a lot of carbohydrates, so you must become very familiar with the contents of your favorite foods. While an average serving of eggs, chicken, fish, and lean meat has none or only 1 gram of carbohydrate in it, a banana has 25 grams, one cup of canned green peas has 31 grams, one baked sweet potato has 36 grams, and a tempting piece of apple pie has 51 grams!

Get in the habit of reading labels—many canned and packaged products now tell you the caloric, protein, and carbohydrate values of their contents. Buy a good calorie and carbohydrate guide. (You can order a good pamphlet, *Nutritive Values of Foods*, published by the U. S. Government Printing Office, Washington, D.C. 20402.) Make lists of the foods you eat and note their calorie and carbohydrate content simultaneously. You'll be on your way to a lifetime of balanced eating, in which you'll choose healthy and nutritious foods that won't load you up with carbohydrates. You can make losing weight a chore, or you can take this opportunity to become educated and enlightened about the foods you eat. When you understand why and how weight is lost, it will make it easier to stick to your prescribed diet and to resume eating in such a "normal" way that you won't add on again those pounds you worked so hard to take off.

Both while you're dieting and once you've established your normal maintenance diet, you might want to consider taking multivitamin and multimineral food supplements daily. There are several good natural products on the market that work in cooperation with nature. For many years now we ourselves have been taking and recommending to our clients Shaklee nutritional vitamin and mineral supplements.

We share the Shaklee basic philosophy: Listen to nature and strive for harmony with nature. Over the years this philosophy has proved invaluable as we've developed a balance and harmony in our own lives through regular exercise and sound nutritional practices.

To establish your own natural harmony, eat nutritionally and form the all-important habit of doing your EXERCISE PLUS exercises three times a week. Practically all our clients have told us at one time or another that one hour spent exercising three times a week actually seemed to decrease rather than increase their appetites. The steady, hour-long set of EXERCISE PLUS routines is the ideal way to control your hunger rather than stimulate it.

Plan your exercise schedule so that you don't eat until at least an hour after you've exercised. "The reason for this," says Dr. Edelstein, "is to give your oxygen supply a chance to stay where it is needed, and not get diverted to your stomach." We'd like to add that you should wait at least an hour after you've eaten to do your EXERCISE PLUS routines. You're going to want your oxygen supply at its maximum to get the most out of your workout.

Remember the basic principles of exercise and diet. Fat cannot be broken down in the body, but it can be used for energy if energy cannot be obtained from some other source. The combination of reduced calories and carbohydrates in the diet with consistent exercise will aid in speeding up weight loss, and will be even more helpful in maintaining it.

Exercise alone will not take off those excess pounds. But combined with proper nutrition, your EXERCISE PLUS routines can make all the difference in the world as you become slimmer, firmer, and healthier—the shape you're meant to be in!

Index

Abdominal muscles, 21
  after childbirth, 22, 106
  EXERCISE PLUS program and, 30–32
  Lying-Down Leg Lifts and, 83
  Neck and Spine Stretch and, 51
  Pelvic Tilt and, 74
  pelvis and lower back region after delivery and, 102
  Pendulum and, 63
  physiology and function of, 30
  protection of backbone and, 22
  rhythmic breathing and, 23–24
  Roll Up and, 54–56
  Rollback and Sit-up Return and, 110
  stress during pregnancy on, 31
Aging process, exercise and, 26
Alcohol consumption, pregnancy and, 42, 43
Amniocentesis, 8
Amniotic sac, growth of, 41
Anesthesia
  changes in use of, 45–46
  during labor, 7–8
Anxiety
  body image and, 37
  reduced by exercise, 17
Appetite loss, postpartum, 103
Arm muscles
  Press and, 87
  Side Bend and, 65
  See also Upper arms

Back
  exercise and, 19, 33–34
  Ring and, 111
  Sitting Leg Lifts and, 80, 81
  See also Backache; Lower back
Back of Thigh Stretch, 98–99
Backache, 21
  abdominal muscle weakness and, 30
  poor posture and, 22
  pregnancy and, 33, 43
Backbone
  abdominal muscles and, 22
  pregnancy and, 21